# The Chart is the Witness

## A Hospice Chaplain's Guide to Documentation as Sacred Practice

Bobby Bressman

GriefBites.org

# The Chart Is the Witness

*A Hospice Chaplain's Guide to Documentation as Sacred Practice*

Dr. Bobby Bressman, D.Min., CGP

Scripture quotations, unless otherwise noted, are drawn from the New International Version (NIV) and the New Living Translation (NLT).

Clinical scenarios throughout this book are composite illustrations built for teaching purposes. Names, ages, diagnoses, and identifying details are fictional and do not represent any actual patient, family, or medical record.

Published by GriefBites | Grief2Growth Foundation

GriefBites.org

First Edition

Formatted with Vellum

# Chapter 1
# Leading From the Limp

Every book like this one has a wound underneath it. I'd rather tell you where mine is than let you go digging for it between the lines. I'm a hospice chaplain, a pastor, and the founder of a bereavement ministry, and I've spent the better part of two decades sitting in rooms where families are losing the person who taught them what love was supposed to look like. I did not arrive at that work in one piece. Nobody does. You arrive broken in a specific place, still walking, permanently changed in your gait.

There's a story in Genesis I've leaned on so many times, in supervision and in the pulpit and in my own late-night wrestling, that I've lost track of which parts are mine and which parts belong to Scripture. Jacob is alone at the river Jabbok. The next morning he has to face a brother he wronged badly enough that he still doesn't know if he's walking toward reconciliation or toward his own death. A man shows up in the dark and wrestles with him until daybreak. Jacob won't let go. Even after his hip is wrenched out of its socket, even after the fight costs him something that will never fully heal, he holds on and says, "I will not let you go unless you bless me." He gets the blessing. He gets a new name — Israel, the one who struggles with God and prevails. Then Genesis tells us something that stops me cold every single time I read it: "So Jacob limped past Peniel as the sun rose."

He got the blessing and kept the limp. Not one, then the other. Both, at the same time, for the rest of his life. That's the truest description of pastoral formation I know, and it is certainly the truest description of my own. I didn't become a hospice chaplain because suffering was an abstraction I found theologically interesting. I have my own Jabbok. I've sat with losses I'm not going to narrate on this page — not to protect a brand, but because some griefs belong to God and to the handful of people who walked through them with me, not to a reading audience. I've lived through the disorientation of pastoral trauma too: the ache of being wounded by the very institution and the very people you gave your life to serve. I have burned out completely. The kind that doesn't respond to a vacation or a pep talk. The kind that makes you wonder if you have anything left to give anyone, ever again.

I tell you this to establish the only credential that actually qualifies a person to write a book like this one. I've walked with a limp long enough to know it's not going away, and I've learned to preach and counsel and lead and chart from inside that limp rather than in spite of it.

Rick Warren has a phrase I've always found clarifying: God never wastes a hurt. I'd push it one step further. He doesn't just refuse to waste our hurts — He builds ministries out of the exact shape of them. GriefBites exists because I needed, more than once, the kind of accompaniment I now try to build for other people. The RESTORE pathway exists because I needed a structure for my own restoration before I had anything to offer someone else's. And this book exists because somewhere in the middle of my own limping, I had a realization about documentation I've never been able to shake.

### GriefBites and the People We Serve

GriefBites has organized itself, as it's grown, around four groups of people.

1. We serve individuals walking through grief directly.
2. We serve pastors and churches trying to companion their congregations through loss without the clinical training a hospice chaplain gets.
3. We serve hospice organizations — the chaplains and bereavement staff inside them, which is who this book is mostly written for.
4. And we serve leaders, pastors and chaplains and hospice executives who are themselves running on fumes while caring for everyone else, often with nobody checking in on how they're doing.

This book is technically about documentation. It is really about the same conviction that runs under everything GriefBites does —

*that grief and burnout are not problems you're supposed to manage privately and silently. They deserve structure and honesty and other people around you.*

Sometimes that structure is a support group. Sometimes it's a coaching relationship. Sometimes, believe it or not, it's a well-written chart note.

I've used the phrase "systems of grace" for years now to describe what I'm actually trying to build, both at GriefBites and in the hospice teams I train. A system of grace isn't a slogan. It's a structure — a workflow, a checklist, a documentation habit, a supervision rhythm — built so that grace doesn't depend entirely on any one chaplain having a good day. I've had bad days. I've walked into rooms running on fumes, grieving something of my own, wondering if I had anything left.

A system of grace is what still lets the patient in that room receive faithful care even when the chaplain delivering it is empty, because the system carries some of the weight the chaplain can't carry alone. Good documentation is one of the most underrated systems of grace our profession has. It doesn't ask you to feel spiritually alive on every visit. It asks you to follow a discipline closely enough that even your worst weeks produce a record good enough to serve the patient, the family, and whoever picks up the case after you.

### What I Owe You

I want you to know something before we go further, because it matters for how you read everything after it. I don't write from a place of having this figured out. I write from a place of having failed at it, repeatedly, in ways both small and consequential, and having slowly and imperfectly built better habits out of those failures. If you're a new chaplain terrified of the blinking cursor in your EMR, I remember that unease. If you're a seasoned chaplain who has drifted into "Provided chaplaincy care. Patient receptive." as your default note, I've written that exact sentence more times than I want to admit — usually on the days I had nothing left for the page because I'd given everything to the room.

One more thing before we get to work. I currently sit in CPEI training, pursuing certification as a Board Certified Chaplain Educator and Supervisor. Which means I'm being formed as a formator, learning how to hand the next generation of chaplains the same disciplines I'm trying to hand you here. That process has sharpened something I want to name plainly: the shift from fixer to witness is not a one-time event. It's a posture you keep choosing, visit after visit, note after note, for the rest of your career. I'm still choosing it. I expect I always will be. My hope isn't that you finish this book with a set of rules you never break. My hope is that you finish it with a theology sturdy enough to make the choosing easier, and habits practical enough to make the choosing sustainable. Even on the hard days. Even with the limp. Especially with the limp.

### FOR REFLECTION

- *Where is your own Jabbok — the wrestling match that shaped how you show up for the dying and their families?*
- *Think of a time your presence with a patient or family had a shorter shelf life than it should have, a time your memory carried something your chart never did. What got lost when that memory faded?*
- *How often do you reach for "Provided chaplaincy care. Patient receptive."? Be honest.*

## Chapter 2

# Why Charting Is Spiritual Care, Not Paperwork

Here's the sentence I've heard in more chaplain offices, more CPE seminar rooms, and more hallway conversations than any other complaint about our discipline: "What we do cannot be written down." I understand the impulse behind it before I push back on it, because something true is buried inside the exaggeration. What happens between a chaplain and a dying patient in a real spiritual encounter does exceed language. The weight in the room when a woman finally says out loud what she's never said to another living soul. The particular quality of silence after a prayer that both of you know mattered. None of that fits neatly into an EMR text box. I've felt the limits of my own vocabulary in front of moments like that more times than I can count.

But the conclusion so many chaplains quietly draw from that true observation is false, and honestly, a little lazy. It goes something like this: *because our work can't be fully captured in writing, we shouldn't try very hard to capture any of it.* That does not follow. And it does real harm to the people we serve.

Most of what we do can be described with precision. What we observed. What the patient said, in their own words. The intervention we chose and why we chose it. What changed, however subtly, in the patient's affect, in the family system, in the spiritual questions sitting on the table. The part that genuinely exceeds language is a sliver of the whole encounter, not the whole encounter. When we hide behind the ineffable to justify a note that reads "*Provided chaplaincy care. Patient receptive,*" We're abandoning our patient to whatever the rest of the team can piece together from vital signs and medication lists. When we do that then the chart has a chaplain-shaped hole in it where the person's soul should be.

Every other discipline on a hospice team documents constantly, almost compulsively, because their professional cultures assume the chart is the primary record of their work.

Nursing narrates. Social work narrates. Even a brief aide note narrates something observable.

Chaplaincy grew up differently, inside a tradition that prized the sanctity of the pastoral encounter above almost everything — confidentiality, presence, the seal of the confessional in some traditions. That instinct isn't wrong. But somewhere along the way, a lot of us let "sacred and confidential" slide quietly into "sacred and therefore unwritten," and those aren't the same thing. You can honor the sanctity of an encounter and still document its shape. Physicians do this constantly with the most intimate conversations imaginable — diagnosis, prognosis, end-of-life decisions — without believing the sanctity of the conversation is compromised by writing it down accurately.

Think about what happens when we don't write.

- The nurse who reads the chart during a crisis visit has no idea this patient told you, three days ago, that she's terrified of dying alone because her mother died alone in a nursing home during COVID.
- The medical director reviewing the case for recertification has no documented evidence spiritual distress is a live issue, so spiritual care quietly falls off the plan of care.
- The social worker following up on a grieving husband has no record you already assessed his isolation last visit and flagged it as a risk.

Your silence in the chart erases the patient's story from the only place the whole team can actually see it. The chart is where they meet this patient when they can't be there in person. Leave that space blank, or fill it with phrases interchangeable enough to describe any patient on any day, and you've failed the very people you claim to be advocating for.

None of this tension is new, and none of it is unique to our field. Every discipline on an interdisciplinary team wrestles with how much detail belongs in a note dozens of people will read under time pressure. But our field has professional standards that settle the question, even when our discomfort with paperwork tries to reopen it. The Association of Professional Chaplains' Standards of Practice are explicit — the chaplain documents

*"in the interdisciplinary treatment/care plan and the medical record in a manner consistent with the care setting"*

and that documentation should communicate assessment, intervention, and outcome in language the whole team can use.

The Joint Commission doesn't ask whether you had a beautiful conversation with a patient. A tracer methodology follows one patient's chart through the system and asks a blunter question:

*did the assessed need lead to a plan, and was that plan actually carried out?*

A chart with no evidence of assessment or follow-through is, in the eyes of a surveyor, evidence the need was never addressed at all. Regardless of what actually happened in the room.

**The History We Inherited**

It helps to understand why our profession's relationship to documentation looks the way it does, because most of us didn't arrive at our resistance out of nowhere. Chaplaincy in America grew up largely inside a pastoral counseling tradition that prized confidentiality above nearly everything, modeled on the seal of confession and the therapeutic privilege of the counseling room. For most of the twentieth century that made sense — a hospital chaplain was often the one person on staff a patient could talk to with an expectation of near-total privacy. That privacy still matters. But healthcare as a whole spent those same decades moving the other direction, toward interdisciplinary teams and shared electronic records and an expectation that every discipline's clinical reasoning be visible to the rest of the team. Chaplaincy's documentation culture didn't fully keep pace. A lot of us are still operating, whether we realize it or not, out of a professional inheritance built for a healthcare system that no longer exists.

The Association of Professional Chaplains has done real work over the past two decades pulling our standards into alignment with the rest of modern healthcare. But standards on paper only change a culture when individual chaplains internalize the reasoning behind them, not just the requirement. That's most of why I wrote this book the way I did. Not as a compliance manual — as an argument for why the shift matters theologically as much as it matters professionally. Chart well because you've come to believe, the way I've come to believe, that it's a genuine act of pastoral faithfulness. Not because a standard told you to.

**Measuring the Immeasurable**

A thoughtful objection worth taking seriously: *isn't there something reductive about trying to measure a spiritual encounter at all? Doesn't fitting a sacred moment into a Data or Action or Plan field flatten something that was never meant to be flattened?*

I share that instinct myself. But the objection rests on a false choice between capturing the encounter with totalizing precision, or refusing to write anything down. There's a third option, and it's been sitting there the whole time. We aren't measuring the sacred the way a lab measures a blood value, claiming to capture its full essence in a number. We're leaving a faithful, partial trace of it, the way a photograph leaves a faithful, partial trace of a person without claiming to capture their entire soul. Nobody objects that a photograph is reductive and therefore not worth taking. We understand instinctively that a photograph isn't the person, and it's still worth keeping, precisely because memory alone isn't enough. A chart note is the same stuff. It doesn't capture the whole encounter. It captures enough of a trace that the encounter isn't lost entirely to time. That's worth doing especially because it will always be incomplete.

So here's the reframe. Documentation isn't the leftover administrative residue of your ministry. It's a continuation of it, extended into a form that outlives the visit. Write a good note and you've made sure this patient's spiritual story doesn't vanish the second you walk out the door. That's not paperwork. Call it what it is.

## FOR REFLECTION

- *Have you ever used "sacred and confidential" as a reason not to document something that was, in fact, safe to write down?*
- *Think of a veteran chaplain you admire whose clinical wisdom you mostly learned by watching them, not reading their notes. What would it have meant for that wisdom to be written down?*
- *Name one piece of spiritual assessment data currently living only in your memory about a patient on your caseload right now.*

# Chapter 3
# The Theology of Documentation — Bearing Witness in the Electronic Age

Professional obligation alone won't carry a chaplain through the tenth note of a long shift. What carries you through is a theology strong enough for the weight of the discipline. So let me build one.

Scripture is saturated with the language of remembering and recording. God tells Israel to write his commands on their doorframes, to build memorial stones at the Jordan so future generations will ask what they mean, to keep a written account of his faithfulness because human memory is porous and gets overwritten by the next crisis. The Psalmist tells God, in Psalm 56, that God himself keeps a record of our sorrows and collects our tears in a bottle. Not because God needs a filing system. Because being truly known means being remembered accurately, in detail, over time.

Chart well and you're participating in an old biblical instinct — the conviction that a person's story deserves to be kept, not lost to tomorrow's forgetting. When charting is done faithfully it becomes an act of faithfulness to the patient in front of you. It's how you keep your promise to remember them the way God remembers them. Specifically. Not generically. Hesed, the Hebrew word usually translated "steadfast love," is never generic in Scripture. It's always covenantal, always attached to a particular relationship and a particular history. Document generically and you're failing, in a small but real way, to extend hesed to the patient in front of you. You're loving a category instead of a person.

**A Trajectory Worth Tracking**

Consider what the chart is actually tracking over the life of a hospice case. In my own framework most patients and families move through a spiritual trajectory with real shape and real stages, even if no two people walk it identically. This borrows from the Old Testament scholar Walter Brueggemann, who described the Psalms as moving through three postures: orientation, disorientation, and new orientation. I've adapted the language for the bedside because I've watched it play out, almost without exception, across every hospice case I've walked alongside.

Patients begin, often, in settled faith. A working theology, simple or sophisticated, that made sense of their life up to now. My life made sense. God was good, or God was distant but predictable, or faith was a background hum I never examined too closely. Then the diagnosis arrives, or hospice gets called, or the decline speeds up, and settled faith cracks. Dis-orientation. Shattered trust. This diagnosis has broken my world, and the theology I was using no longer holds the weight I'm putting on it. That is not a crisis to fear or rush past. Biblically, it's the beginning of lament. It is the same movement across the Psalms of complaint, where the psalmist names the brokenness honestly before God instead of performing a faith he doesn't currently feel.

Let me make lament concrete, because I think chaplains benefit from seeing the actual shape of it rather than a general impression. Take Psalm 13. It opens in raw complaint: "*How long, Lord? Will you forget me forever? How long will you hide your face from me?*" That's not polite prayer. That's a believer accusing God, directly, of abandonment. The psalm moves into petition — specific requests: "*Look on me and answer, Lord my God. Give light to my eyes.*" And it closes, almost abruptly, in praise: "*But I trust in your unfailing love; my heart rejoices in your salvation.*" Notice what didn't happen between the complaint and the praise. The circumstances didn't change. Nothing in the text says the crisis resolved. What changed was posture that moved from accusation to trust and that shift happened inside the lament, not instead of it.

When I sit with a patient moving through Dis-orientation, I'm listening for that same shape, trying to help them access all three movements instead of getting stuck in the first or performing the third too early. A chaplain who only offers reassurance is trying to skip a family straight to Psalm 13's last line without letting them say verse one out loud first. It rarely works. When it seems to work, it usually produces exactly the thin, generic peace that collapses the moment real grief revisits the room.

If our documentation only ever records "patient verbalized peace," we've erased the shattering actually happening — and erased the very material God tends to use to bring someone toward something deeper.

This is also where hesed does its heaviest lifting. The psalmist in Psalm 13 can move all the way to praise in the middle of an unresolved crisis because hesed doesn't depend on the crisis resolving. It depends on the character of the One being trusted. Chaplains sometimes unconsciously believe our presence should mirror only the praise movement, that our job is to usher patients toward peaceful resolution and that lingering in complaint or petition is some kind of pastoral failure. Hesed frees us from that pressure. If God's steadfast love doesn't require the crisis to resolve before it's real, our presence doesn't require the patient to arrive at peace before it's valuable. We can sit inside someone's complaint for as long as they need us there, trusting hesed is already operating in that room whether or not anyone names it out loud.

Given honest companionship rather than premature reassurance, many patients move through shattered trust toward a third place: Re-orientation. Not a return to old settled faith. A new, tested reliance on God that's been through the fire and come out different. This is the territory the posttraumatic growth research describes —

*suffering, held well, can produce genuine psychological and spiritual development alongside the damage, not instead of it.*

Richard Tedeschi and Lawrence Calhoun, who coined the term in the 1990s, identified five domains where this growth tends to show up:

- a greater appreciation for life,
- warmer relationships,
- a felt sense of new possibilities,
- a deepened sense of personal strength,
- and spiritual or existential change.

I keep those domains loosely in mind during a Re-orientation conversation, not as a checklist to impose but as listening posts. A patient who tells you the diagnosis made them call an estranged sister for the first time in a decade is describing relational growth. A patient who says they've started noticing sunsets in a way they never used to is describing a new appreciation for life. None of it requires the patient to use my language, or Tedeschi and Calhoun's language, or even explicitly religious language.

*Our job is recognizing the domain when we hear it and writing it down with enough specificity that its significance survives the retelling.*

Growth, in this research, doesn't erase the pain. It exists alongside it. A patient can be experiencing real spiritual growth and still be furious they're dying at fifty-eight. Both things are true, and our documentation should be able to hold both.

It's also the territory Job describes at the end of his long argument with God: "*My ears had heard of you, but now my eyes have seen you.*" That sentence is the hinge of the whole book. Job doesn't get his questions answered. He doesn't get his children back. What he gets is an encounter that moves his knowledge of God from secondhand report to firsthand sight. That's the emotional peak we're listening for in every hospice room, and it's the peak our documentation should be trained to notice when it happens. Chart the shift from "I've made my peace with God" to "I don't understand why God let this happen" to "I feel him closer now than I ever did before I got sick," and you're not filling a field. You're handing the interdisciplinary team, and eventually the bereavement team, a map of this specific soul's journey — one that will matter enormously when it comes time to grieve them.

There's a practical reason this matters to people who aren't chaplains at all. A nurse managing pain, a social worker assessing a family's coping capacity, a bereavement counselor planning a risk-stratified follow-up schedule — none of them are trained theologians and none of them need to be, once you've translated this into your documentation. Write that a patient has moved from settled faith into shattered trust, and you've given a nurse a plausible explanation for why that patient's pain reporting got harder to manage this week (spiritual distress reliably amplifies physical suffering; we'll come back to that directly in one of the encounters ahead). You've given a social worker language for why a family that seemed to be coping fine last month is struggling this month. You've given a bereavement counselor a running start on a risk assessment that would otherwise start from zero.

### Anti-Transactional Faith

A great deal of popular American Christianity, even when it doesn't say so out loud, runs on transactional logic: if I do good, God protects me. If I have enough faith, I won't suffer, or won't suffer long. Job's friends are the great biblical case study in this logic, and the whole book exists to dismantle it. Job has done nothing to deserve his suffering. His friends spend chapter after chapter insisting he must have, because the alternative — that God allows devastating suffering to fall on the faithful for reasons that aren't punishment — is theologically unbearable to them. But it's the truth Job has to make peace with, and it's the truth every dying patient eventually has to make peace with too, whether or not they have the vocabulary for it.

Our job isn't defending the transactional logic on God's behalf. Our job is walking people out of it, gently, toward the faith Job arrives at — rooted not in "if I do good, God protects me" but in "you are loved before you perform, and you remain loved regardless of the outcome." That sentence — you are loved before you perform — is the most pastorally load-bearing line in this book. It belongs in your prayers at the bedside. It belongs, in its own clinical register, in your documentation, whenever you chart a patient moving away from a transactional theology of suffering and toward something anchored in grace.

### The Chaplain's Own Trajectory

One more thing worth naming before we move past the theology and into the actual notes. The Orientation, Dis-orientation, Re-orientation pattern isn't just something that happens to our patients. It happens to us, across a career, and often across a single hard week. I've watched new chaplains arrive at this work with a settled, almost tidy theology of suffering, the kind that survives a classroom but hasn't yet been tested by a bedside. Then a case comes along that breaks it. A child. A death that happens badly, despite everyone's best effort. A family that turns on each other in the room. And the chaplain's own settled faith cracks in exactly the way Chapter Three describes happening to patients, because chaplains are not exempt from the disorientation we're trained to walk other people through.

I mention this because it changes how you should read everything else in this book. I am not writing from Re-orientation as a permanent, achieved state, immune to further disorientation. Nobody gets to stay there. I've cycled through all three postures more times than I can count, sometimes within the same month, sometimes because of a single case that stayed with me longer than it should have. What Re-orientation actually offers isn't immunity from future disorientation. It's a track record. Evidence, accumulated over enough cycles, that disorientation doesn't have the final word, even when it feels, in the moment, like it might.

This matters for your documentation practice specifically, not just your inner life, because a chaplain in acute disorientation is at real risk of two opposite documentation failures.

- The first is going quiet — the notes get thinner, more generic, more "provided chaplaincy care," because the chaplain doesn't have the internal resources that week to write with real specificity.
- The second, less obvious, is overcompensating with notes that perform a spiritual confidence the chaplain doesn't actually feel, papering over their own crisis with theological language borrowed rather than lived.

Both are worth watching for in yourself, and both are exactly the kind of pattern a good supervisor or peer group can catch before it becomes habitual. If you notice your own notes going thin, or noticeably more polished than usual in a way that feels performative, that's worth naming out loud to someone before it becomes the water you swim in without seeing it.

**Writing as if Someone Is Reading**

One more layer, more sobering than the rest, and I'd be doing you a disservice to leave it out. Families read these notes. State surveyors read these notes. In the worst cases, attorneys and courts read these notes.

I'm not telling you that to make you anxious or turn your presence into a defensive crouch. I'm telling you because integrity and accuracy are theological commitments, not just risk-management tactics. Scripture has harsh words for false witness and careless speech, and a chart entry is a form of testimony. Write as though the patient, the family, your supervisor, and possibly an attorney are looking over your shoulder. Not because you're afraid of them. Because you want the record to hold up under any scrutiny, precisely because it's true.

Paint the picture. Write what you saw. Write what was said, in the person's own words where you can. Write your clinical reasoning plainly enough that another chaplain could pick this note up in six months and understand exactly where this patient is on their journey, and why you intervened the way you did. That's not defensive charting. That's honest charting. And honest charting is, itself, an act of faithfulness.

**FOR REFLECTION**

- *Where would you place a current patient on the Orientation, Dis-orientation, Re-orientation trajectory right now — and what specific language from your last visit supports that placement?*
- *Where have you operated out of a transactional theology of suffering, and what moved you, if anything has, toward something more anchored in grace?*
- *Reread your last three notes. Would a stranger know this patient's specific fears and specific words, or could these notes describe almost anyone?*

# Chapter 4
# Documentation Frameworks — Finding Your Format

There is no one correct documentation model, and any chaplain educator who tells you otherwise is overselling their favorite. What every hospice chaplain needs is a format, used consistently, because consistency is what lets the rest of the interdisciplinary team find what they need without hunting for it inside your prose every single time. Here are four models I've used, taught, or watched work well in different hospice systems, so you can choose — or your agency can choose for you — with your eyes open.

**DAROP: Data, Action, Results, Observations, Plan**

Developed by Dr. Saul Ebema, this model has become a favorite in hospice settings because its structure maps cleanly onto the language the Conditions of Participation expect: an assessment of need **(Data)**, a documented intervention **(Action)**, a measurable outcome **(Results, Observations)**, and forward-looking care **(Plan)**. I like it for newer chaplains because the acronym itself functions as a checklist. Can't fill in all five letters? You probably haven't finished thinking through the visit. A one-line skeleton might look like this —

*Data: patient tearful, states fear of dying alone.*
*Action: validated fear, offered presence and prayer.*
*Results: affect calmed, patient thanked chaplain.*
*Observations: unresolved anticipatory grief, low family support.*
*Plan: weekly visits, SW referral for support system.*

Not a finished note. But notice how it forces you through the whole clinical arc in five short beats.

**The Memorial Hermann Five-Part Model**

**Reason for Visit, Interventions, Outcomes, Assessment, Plan**. Many chaplaincy educators consider this the gold standard, and I understand why. It front-loads the "why was I even in the room" question, forcing you to articulate your clinical rationale before you describe what you did. It separates Outcomes from Assessment, a subtlety worth sitting with — outcomes are what you observed change (or didn't) during the visit itself, while assessment is your ongoing clinical judgment about where the patient sits spiritually, drawing on more than just today. Takes a little more discipline to use well. Produces some of the richest documentation I've read in twenty years of hospice work. I recommend it to chaplains further along in their formation who want their charting to carry the same clinical weight as a physician's or social worker's assessment.

**SOAP: Subjective, Objective, Assessment, Plan**

The format the rest of the medical team already speaks fluently, which is the whole advantage. If your EMR pushes every discipline toward a shared SOAP template, or your IDG is heavy on nursing and physician voices trained to think in SOAP, this lets your note sit naturally alongside everyone else's instead of looking like a foreign document dropped into a medical chart. The tradeoff: SOAP wasn't built with spiritual assessment in mind, so you'll feel the seams. Spiritual "objective" data is a stranger concept than physical objective data, and you'll need your own convention for what counts. I train chaplains using SOAP to treat direct quotes, observed affect, ritual participation, and religious artifacts in the room — a Bible on the nightstand, a rosary in a patient's hand — as their objective data. Not vital signs. Still observable, which is the actual standard.

**Spiritual AIM**

**Assessment, Intervention, Outcome**, mapped to domains like Self-Worth or Community and Belonging. If your hospice uses the Spiritual AIM screening tool out of the Rush University tradition, this lets your documentation speak the same domain language as your intake screening. This provides real continuity from admission through the whole length of stay. A patient screened with a "meaning" deficit at intake should show up in your ongoing notes with interventions and outcomes mapped to that same domain, so anyone reviewing the case can trace the spiritual care plan from first assessment to most recent visit without translation. This one asks the most of you theologically, because it requires thinking in domains rather than narrative. Agencies that adopt it well report some of the most sophisticated interdisciplinary conversations about spiritual care I've seen anywhere.

**One Encounter, Four Formats**

Description sometimes teaches less than demonstration. Here's the same brief encounter, charted four different ways, so you can see how much of the underlying clinical content stays constant even as the container changes.

**The encounter: This chaplain visited Mrs. G., 72, metastatic breast cancer, at a routine follow-up visit. Patient stated, "I keep asking God why, and I don't get an answer, and honestly I'm getting tired of asking."**

**Patient's daughter was present and appeared uncomfortable with her mother's statement, changing the subject twice. This chaplain validated the patient's exhaustion with unanswered prayer, gently named that her daughter's discomfort might be worth naming between the two of them, and offered to facilitate that conversation at a future visit if patient wished.**

**DAROP — DATA:** Patient stated, "I keep asking God why, and I don't get an answer, and honestly I'm getting tired of asking." Daughter present, visibly uncomfortable, redirected conversation twice during the statement. ACTION: This chaplain validated patient's spiritual exhaustion and named the daughter's discomfort as a potential topic for future facilitated conversation. RESULTS: Patient stated relief at having the exhaustion named plainly rather than corrected. Daughter did not respond verbally. OBSERVATIONS: Patient in active spiritual struggle regarding unanswered prayer; family system shows early signs of discomfort with patient's honest lament. PLAN: This chaplain will offer a facilitated conversation between patient and daughter at next visit if patient remains interested.

**Memorial Hermann — REASON FOR VISIT:** Routine follow-up spiritual care visit. INTERVENTIONS: This chaplain validated patient's exhaustion with unanswered prayer without offering premature theological resolution, and named the daughter's visible discomfort as worth addressing directly between them. OUTCOMES: Patient expressed relief at having her exhaustion acknowledged rather than corrected; daughter's discomfort was named but not yet processed. ASSESSMENT: Patient is in an active, unresolved season of lament regarding unanswered prayer; the family system, represented here by the daughter, has not yet caught up to the patient's willingness to sit honestly in that lament. PLAN: This chaplain will offer a facilitated conversation between patient and daughter at the next visit, contingent on patient's continued interest.

**SOAP — SUBJECTIVE:** Patient stated, "I keep asking God why, and I don't get an answer, and honestly I'm getting tired of asking." OBJECTIVE: Daughter present, changed subject twice during patient's statement, did not make verbal response to this chaplain's reflection. ASSESSMENT: Patient experiencing active spiritual distress consistent with unanswered lament; family discomfort with patient's honesty is an emerging dynamic worth monitoring. PLAN: This chaplain will offer to facilitate a conversation between patient and daughter regarding the daughter's discomfort at a future visit.

**Spiritual AIM (Domain:** Meaning) — ASSESSMENT: Patient is actively wrestling with a perceived absence of divine response to sustained prayer, expressing fatigue with the practice of asking without answer; daughter's discomfort suggests a family system not yet aligned with patient's honest spiritual struggle. INTERVENTION: This chaplain validated the patient's exhaustion without offering resolution, and named the family dynamic gently in the room. OUTCOME: Patient reported relief; family dynamic remains unaddressed and will require further attention. PLAN: This chaplain will continue to track this domain and will offer facilitated family conversation at patient's readiness.

Same eleven seconds of patient speech. Four different clinical vocabularies wrapped around it. Notice, though, that the actual clinical content barely moves — the patient's exhaustion, the daughter's discomfort, the plan to potentially facilitate a conversation between them, all survive the translation intact. That's the whole argument of this chapter in miniature. The framework is a container, not a constraint on what you're able to say. Master any one of these well enough and you'll find yourself able to think in all four, which matters the day you change agencies, or the day your current agency changes its EMR template out from under you, which happens more often than any of us would like.

### Choosing for Your Team

If you're the person tasked with actually picking a model, here's the practical version. If your EMR already has a built-in chaplaincy template, start there — fighting your own software to force a different framework onto it costs more in friction than it gains in theoretical purity. If your team is full of chaplains in their first two years? Lean DAROP; the built-in checklist quality does real pedagogical work while habits are still forming. Experienced team, agency culture that already values rich narrative documentation? Memorial Hermann will reward that maturity. IDG dominated by nursing and physician voices who think natively in SOAP? Match their language and cut the translation friction at exactly the moments spiritual care needs to be heard clearly. Agency invested in Spiritual AIM at intake? Use it for ongoing documentation too. The continuity from admission to final visit is worth more than anything else on this list.

Build the decision into new-hire orientation explicitly, not as an aside. I've watched agencies buy excellent training materials and fail to enforce the format after the first ninety days, at which point every chaplain drifts back to whatever they learned in CPE or their last job. Consistency is a leadership discipline as much as a personal one.

None of these models is theologically superior to the others, What matters more than which model you choose is that your agency chooses one and holds to it. A hospice where every chaplain runs a different personal system produces a chart that reads like four languages spoken in the same room, and that inconsistency is exactly what a surveyor, or a plaintiff's attorney, notices first. In the chapters ahead, I've rotated through all four models on purpose, so you can watch each one earn its keep against real material. The clinical and theological content underneath stays constant even as the container changes. That's the whole point.

## FOR REFLECTION

- *Which of these four models does your agency use, if any? What has the inconsistency, if there is any, cost your team on a handoff?*
- *If you could choose freely, which model fits how your mind naturally organizes a visit?*

# Chapter 5
# The Original Eight Encounters — Charting Examples With Commentary

This is the working heart of the book. Eight encounters drawn from the rhythm of a hospice chaplain's caseload, each with a fully written note, a short explanation of why the note works, and a CPE learning edge connecting the discipline back to your own formation. I've never met a chaplain who charted well who didn't first learn to observe well, and observation is exactly what verbatim work trains. I've rotated through all four frameworks from the last chapter so you can watch them earn their keep against real material.

A word on how to move through this chapter: don't read all eight back to back in one sitting, tempting as that is. Read one, sit with the commentary long enough to notice your own reaction to it, work through the learning edge honestly, then move to the next. These notes reward slow reading more than fast reading, and slowing down is where most of the actual formation in this book happens.

# Scenario A: Initial Spiritual Assessment (Home Visit) — DAROP Format

**Patient: Mrs. Helen M., 78-year-old female, CHF (congestive heart failure)**

**DATA:** Patient alert and oriented, seated in recliner with oxygen in place with a nasal cannula, breathing comfortably at rest. Husband James present in the home. This chaplain conducted the initial spiritual assessment visit. When asked how she was making sense of her diagnosis, patient stated, "I've made my peace with God, but I'm worried about Jimmy when I'm gone." Patient identified as lifelong Methodist, described a settled and consistent faith history, and did not present with acute spiritual distress regarding her own death. Her stated concern centered entirely on her husband's future wellbeing.

**ACTION:** This chaplain validated the appropriateness and depth of her concern for her husband, naming that love for another person outliving our own fear is itself a spiritual strength. At patient's request, this chaplain read Psalm 23 aloud and closed with prayer that named both her peace and her worry honestly before God. This chaplain also engaged James directly during the visit, observing his affect and asking about his own support system, and noted signs consistent with social isolation, including his statement that "it's just been the two of us for a long time now."

**RESULTS:** Patient's affect brightened visibly during the reading of Psalm 23 and she stated, "That's my favorite one, always has been." She thanked this chaplain for taking her concern for James seriously rather than redirecting the conversation back to her own prognosis.

**OBSERVATIONS:** Patient presents with settled faith and low spiritual distress regarding her own death. Primary spiritual and psychosocial concern is anticipatory grief and caregiver risk for surviving spouse. James presents with early indicators of social isolation warranting interdisciplinary follow-up.

**PLAN:** This chaplain will continue routine visits every two weeks per plan of care. This chaplain referred James's isolation risk to the social worker for caregiver support assessment and will personally follow up with James individually within one week, separate from a patient visit, to begin building rapport ahead of anticipated bereavement.

**Why This Works:** The note doesn't just record that a prayer happened. It records the reasoning behind it — why Psalm 23, what the patient's response revealed, how that response confirmed the chaplain's read of the room. It also catches something a lot of chaplains miss on a first visit: it assesses the caregiver, not only the patient. Hospice has always treated the family as the unit of care, and this note proves it in a way a surveyor, or a social worker picking up the case tomorrow, can act on immediately. And the note resists manufacturing distress that isn't there. Helen genuinely has settled faith about her own death. A weaker chaplain, primed to expect distress, might have pushed past that reality hunting for something more dramatic to write down.

**CPE Learning Edge:** A good early test of use of self. A newer chaplain, uncomfortable with a patient's calm acceptance of her own death, might unconsciously push the conversation deeper into Helen's mortality, chasing a catharsis she didn't need because the chaplain needed to feel useful. Verbatim work trains you to catch that pull before it hijacks the visit. Here the better move was following the patient's own lead toward her husband, which required setting aside a private agenda about what a "meaningful" assessment visit is supposed to look like. If you're ever disappointed that a patient doesn't need deep spiritual processing, bring that disappointment to supervision. It usually says more about the chaplain's need to be needed than about the patient.

# Scenario B: The Stoic Patient (Follow-Up Visit) — Memorial Hermann Five-Part Model

**Patient: Mr. C., 68-year-old male, COPD (chronic obstructive pulmonary disease)**

**REASON FOR VISIT:** Routine follow-up spiritual care visit. Wife Doris reports patient is minimally verbal about his emotional state, consistently responding "I'm fine" to direct questions, though she has observed nighttime anxiety including restlessness and difficulty settling for sleep.

**INTERVENTIONS:** Given patient's established pattern of deflecting direct emotional inquiry, this chaplain used indirect narrative questioning, asking about past hardships the patient has weathered rather than asking about his current feelings directly. Patient volunteered a story about the 2019 drought and the loss of a significant portion of his cattle herd, describing the financial and personal toll of that season. When asked how he got through it, patient stated, "You just get up the next day." This chaplain did not press for further emotional disclosure or attempt to draw an explicit parallel between that loss and his current diagnosis. This chaplain affirmed the resilience embedded in his statement and offered a brief silent prayer at the patient's side, honoring his preference for minimal verbal processing.

**OUTCOMES:** Patient remained physically present and attentive throughout the silent prayer, eyes closed, hands folded, a departure from his usual restlessness during chaplain visits. He did not verbally acknowledge the prayer afterward but nodded once when this chaplain said, "I'll keep sitting with you, however that looks for you."

**ASSESSMENT:** Patient's coping style is consistent with a stoic, self-reliant orientation shaped by a lifetime of practical resilience. His verbal minimization ("I'm fine") likely coexists with genuine underlying anxiety, evidenced by Doris's report of nighttime symptoms. Not a contradiction — the stated affect and the somatic affect are simply tracking on different channels. Direct emotional confrontation is unlikely to be therapeutic here and may increase his guardedness.

**PLAN:** This chaplain will continue brief, twice-monthly, presence-focused visits without pressing for verbal catharsis. This chaplain will assess Doris's caregiver stress at the next visit, as her role interpreting and managing his unspoken anxiety alone is a significant burden.

**Why This Works:** The note resists a temptation every chaplain faces with a stoic patient: pathologizing the stoicism as denial that needs breaking through. Instead the assessment names his coping style accurately and respectfully, and the plan honors it rather than working against it. Clinically sound and theologically sound at the same time — presence doesn't require confession to be real. There's a quiet theological claim buried in this note too, that God can be present in a silent, wordless prayer beside a man who will never narrate his fear out loud, and the chaplain's job isn't extracting a confession God doesn't require.

**CPE Learning Edge:** A countertransference checkpoint. Grew up with a parent who never talked about their feelings? A patient like Mr. C. can activate old frustration in you before you notice it happening. A chaplain unaware of that pull might chart the visit as a "failure to engage" or push the next visit toward extraction instead of presence. Writing an honest assessment — one that separates what the patient needs from what would satisfy the chaplain's own discomfort with silence — is exactly the discipline verbatim work builds. Does the word "failure" ever show up in your notes about patients who simply cope differently than you do?

# Scenario C: Family Caregiver in Distress (PRN Visit) — SOAP Format

**Patient's Daughter: Susan, 52-year-old female, daughter of Mrs. A., 84-year-old female, dementia**

**SUBJECTIVE:** This chaplain was called for a PRN visit after Susan, primary caregiver for her mother, was found crying in the hallway by nursing staff. Upon arrival, Susan stated, "I can't do this anymore. I don't know how much longer I can keep doing this." She described exhaustion, guilt over feeling resentful of her caregiving role, and a sense of spiritual disconnection, stating she is Catholic but has not been able to attend Mass in several months due to caregiving demands.

**OBJECTIVE:** Susan was tearful, speech pressured, sitting hunched with her arms wrapped around herself in the hallway outside her mother's room. She made intermittent eye contact and her hands trembled visibly during the conversation.

**ASSESSMENT:** Caregiver presenting with acute emotional distress consistent with caregiver burnout, compounded by spiritual disconnection related to prolonged absence from her faith community and its sacramental life. No safety concerns identified for Susan herself. This chaplain assesses her distress as an appropriate and expected response to a sustained caregiving burden, not a pathological reaction.

**PLAN:** This chaplain normalized the overwhelm Susan is experiencing as a common and legitimate response to long-term caregiving, not a personal or spiritual failure. This chaplain explored available spiritual resources with Susan, who expressed a specific longing for the sacrament of communion given her inability to attend Mass. This chaplain offered prayer at Susan's request. This chaplain contacted the hospice social worker to initiate a respite care assessment for Susan and contacted Susan's parish to arrange a communion visit from her priest. This chaplain will return within twenty-four hours to follow up, and the social worker will separately assess respite options.

**Why This Works:** The note draws a clean line between what the chaplain assessed (a legitimate, expected caregiver response, not a crisis) and what the chaplain did about it (normalization, spiritual resource activation, referral). It shows real interdisciplinary coordination without the chaplain trying to solve every problem solo. Notice the plan for Susan is separated from the plan for the patient — Susan is, in this moment, also a person receiving spiritual care in her own right, and the chart reflects that. It's a small but important theological move: hospice care, at its best, refuses to treat the caregiver as merely instrumental to the patient's comfort. Susan's own soul matters here, independent of her usefulness to her mother's care.

**CPE Learning Edge:** A PRN crisis visit is where the fixer instinct gets loudest. Susan is crying in a hallway. Everything in your training before CPE probably told you to fix that crying. The formation work is learning to sit in the hallway without needing to make the crying stop, trusting that presence and appropriate referrals are the intervention. Check your own note for language that reveals a fixer posture. Did you write "resolved her distress" anywhere? You shouldn't have, because you didn't, and you weren't supposed to.

# Scenario D: Spiritual Distress / Guilt and Shame — DAROP Format

**Patient: Mr. R., 71-year-old male, end-stage liver disease**

**DATA:** This chaplain visited Mr. R. at his stated request through nursing. Patient appeared visibly distressed, stating, "God can't forgive what I've done." Upon gentle inquiry, patient disclosed a fifteen-year estrangement from his adult children, which he attributes to his prior struggles with alcoholism. Patient expressed profound guilt and shame and made a statement consistent with a passive death wish, stating, "Maybe it would be better if I just didn't wake up one of these mornings." Patient denied any active plan, intent, or means, and denied any history of suicide attempts.

**ACTION:** This chaplain conducted a direct safety assessment, clarifying with the patient that his statement reflected a wish for the pain to end rather than an active intention to end his own life; patient confirmed this and denied any current plan or intent. This chaplain validated the depth of his regret without minimizing it, and offered a ritual of absolution grounded in the patient's own Christian tradition, naming to him directly, "Your worth was given to you before you did anything right, and it was never taken away by anything you did wrong." With patient's explicit permission, this chaplain contacted his estranged adult son by phone to explore his openness to reconciliation contact.

**RESULTS:** Patient wept during the ritual of absolution and stated afterward, "I haven't heard anything like that in a long time." His son, when contacted, expressed cautious openness to a phone call with his father, stating he needed a few days to consider it.

**OBSERVATIONS:** Patient is experiencing acute spiritual distress rooted in guilt, shame, and estrangement, with an associated passive death wish assessed as low acuity given absence of plan, intent, or means. This presentation is clinically significant and warrants close monitoring alongside spiritual intervention focused on grace, forgiveness, and reconciliation.

**PLAN:** This chaplain will visit twice weekly to continue safety monitoring and to facilitate potential reconciliation with his son as that process unfolds. This chaplain notified the RN case manager and will present this case at the next IDG meeting given the passive death wish, to ensure the full team is aware and coordinated on monitoring.

**Why This Works:** This note does what a lot of chaplains are afraid to do. It documents a passive death wish plainly and clinically, without overreacting or minimizing. It separates the safety assessment from the theological intervention, which protects the patient and the chaplain both, and shows the IDG notification a disclosure like this requires. The absolution ritual is described specifically enough — the actual words spoken — that another chaplain, or a supervisor, could understand exactly what theological move was made and why. That line, your worth was given to you before you did anything right, is the anti-transactional theology from Chapter Three landing at an actual bedside. Worth memorizing.

**CPE Learning Edge:** Passive death wishes surface a chaplain's own anxiety about mortality, and about being the last line of defense in a moment that feels enormously consequential. This is where supervision matters most. Before you chart an encounter like this, ask yourself honestly: did I do a real safety assessment, or did I do a safety assessment that let me feel reassured enough to move on? Verbatim work trains you to slow down exactly these moments. Your documentation should show that same slowed-down rigor, not a rushed reassurance the danger has passed.

# Scenario E: Nonverbal / Unresponsive Patient — DAROP Format

**Patient: Mrs. T., 83-year-old female, senile degeneration (advanced dementia)**

**DATA:** Patient nonverbal since approximately 2022 per chart history, bedbound, currently exhibiting Cheyne-Stokes respirations. Per family report and chart history, patient was a lifelong Methodist and served for many years as her church's choir director. This chaplain entered the room, introduced self by name and role despite patient's unresponsive presentation, and held her hand throughout the visit.

**ACTION:** This chaplain sang "Amazing Grace" quietly at the bedside, selected specifically because of the patient's documented history as a choir director, on the premise that hearing and musical memory often persist even in advanced unresponsiveness. This chaplain offered a prayer of commendation and, per the patient's advance directive on file requesting anointing, anointed her forehead with holy oil.

**RESULTS:** Patient's respiratory pattern did not visibly change during the visit. This chaplain observed a brief, subtle softening of the patient's facial musculature during the hymn, though this chaplain notes this observation cautiously, as reflexive facial movement in this clinical state cannot be reliably interpreted as conscious response.

**OBSERVATIONS:** Patient remains unresponsive and is not able to participate verbally or behaviorally in spiritual assessment. Spiritual care in this stage is oriented toward presence, sensory comfort consistent with the patient's known history and preferences, and support of the family system rather than direct patient engagement.

**PLAN:** This chaplain will continue weekly bedside presence visits. This chaplain will coordinate with nursing and CNA staff to include familiar hymns during routine care activities, given the patient's documented history and likely comfort from music. Family will be notified promptly by nursing per protocol as active dying progresses, with this chaplain available for bedside support at that time.

**Why This Works:** Honest, careful language around a genuinely uncertain clinical observation. It reports the facial movement without overclaiming what it means, and that restraint matters for credibility, and it matters theologically too — we don't need to manufacture evidence of a response to justify the value of the visit. The visit was valuable because it honored the whole person, informed by her history, whether or not she could register it consciously.

**CPE Learning Edge:** Nonverbal patients are where fixer-to-witness becomes most visible in your own writing, because there's nothing to fix and nothing to extract. No patient quotes to lean on. No dialogue to analyze. What you have instead is observational presence — what you noticed, what you chose, why. A chaplain still stuck in fixer mode will pad a note like this one with vague spiritual language to make the visit sound more eventful than it was. A chaplain who has actually internalized witness will write plainly: I was here, I attended to this specific person's specific history, and here is exactly what I observed.

# Scenario F: Death Vigil / Actively Dying — Memorial Hermann Five-Part Model

**Patient: Mr. L., 76-year-old male, metastatic lung cancer**

**REASON FOR VISIT:** This chaplain was called to the bedside during active dying. Patient unresponsive, mottling present in lower extremities, breathing seemed irregular with increasing periods of apnea. Wife Margaret and adult children present at bedside. Family specifically requested that this chaplain "pray him home."

**INTERVENTIONS:** This chaplain affirmed for the family that hearing is widely understood to be the last sense to fade, and encouraged each family member present to speak directly to Mr. L. and say what they needed to say, rather than speaking about him in the room. This chaplain offered a prayer of commendation at the family's request, entrusting Mr. L. into God's care by name. Following the prayer, this chaplain provided approximately twenty minutes of unhurried silence at the bedside, remaining present without initiating further conversation, allowing the family space to sit with their own goodbyes.

**OUTCOMES:** Each family member spoke individually to Mr. L. during the visit. Margaret, his wife, stated afterward, "I think he heard us. I really think he did." The family's affect shifted visibly from anxious activity at the start of the visit to a settled, quiet presence by its conclusion.

**ASSESSMENT:** Family is coping with anticipatory grief through active engagement and ritual participation, which appears to be serving them well. No indicators of complicated grief risk identified at this time, though this will be reassessed at bereavement follow-up given the intensity of the vigil.

**PLAN:** This chaplain will remain available on-call to the family through the remainder of the dying process. Per standard protocol, bereavement will make initial contact with the family within forty-eight hours following the patient's death.

**Why This Works:** A high-emotion encounter captured without a single sentimental phrase. The specific intervention — encouragement to speak directly, the prayer, the deliberate silence — sits next to a specific observable outcome — the family's own words, the visible shift in affect. It sets bereavement up for success by flagging what to watch for at follow-up, rather than treating the vigil as a closed chapter.

**CPE Learning Edge:** One of the most physically and spiritually demanding encounters a chaplain has, and it's tempting to let your own emotional experience of the room bleed into the note. How moving it was. How sacred it felt to you. Resist that. The note belongs to the patient and family's experience, not yours. Your own response belongs in supervision, in your own processing, maybe in a verbatim you bring to your CPE group. Keeping that line clear in your charting is one of the clearest markers of formation I know how to name.

# Scenario G: Bereavement Follow-Up (Phone Call, Three Weeks Post-Death) — SOAP Format

**Contact: James M., 80-year-old male, surviving spouse of Mrs. Helen M. (Scenario A)**

**SUBJECTIVE:** This chaplain conducted a scheduled bereavement follow-up phone call with James, three weeks following Helen's death. James reported eating one meal daily, down from his usual pattern, and sleeping four to five hours nightly with the assistance of prescribed sleep medication. He stated, "The house is too quiet." When asked about his spiritual life since Helen's death, James stated that his prayers "feel like talking to the ceiling."

**OBJECTIVE:** James's voice was flat throughout the call, with longer pauses than in prior conversations. He did not initiate conversation topics and required prompting to elaborate.

**ASSESSMENT:** James's stated diminished appetite, reduced sleep, and stated spiritual disconnection are consistent with a normal, expected grief response at this early stage of bereavement, though the combination of symptoms represents a meaningful escalation from his risk level at Helen's time of death. This chaplain assesses his risk level as elevated from moderate to high, because of appetite change, sleep disruption, and spiritual disconnection occurring together.

**PLAN:** This chaplain normalized James's experience of spiritual disconnection explicitly, naming that feeling distant from God in grief is a well-documented and common experience, not evidence of spiritual failure or abandonment. This chaplain will call again in two weeks to reassess, and will consult with the bereavement coordinator regarding a possible MSW referral given the elevated risk profile, particularly the appetite and sleep changes.

**Why This Works:** A good model for charting a risk escalation clearly enough that whoever touches this file next — another chaplain, a bereavement counselor, an MSW — knows immediately why the tier changed and what drove it. It also shows good theological instinct. James's line about prayer feeling like talking to the ceiling isn't treated as a crisis to correct. It's an accurate description of the Dis-orientation stage, worth naming honestly instead of smoothing over.

**CPE Learning Edge:** Bereavement calls, done by phone without the visual cues of an in-person visit, train a very specific kind of listening — tone, pacing, pauses as data in themselves, not just content. The Objective section here relies entirely on vocal and behavioral observations because that's all the medium allows. Worth naming explicitly in supervision: what do you lose, and what do you gain, when the encounter has no face to read?

# Scenario H: IDG Communication and Team Collaboration

***Sample Verbal IDG Report:***

*"I want to flag three things from spiritual care this week. First, on Mr. D.'s case, I'm seeing a strong connection between his spiritual and existential anxiety and his reported pain control. He's told me directly that when his fear about what happens after death spikes, his pain feels worse and less responsive to his current morphine regimen, even without a change in his physical condition. I don't think this is a dosing problem; I think it's an anxiety amplification problem with a spiritual root, and I'd like nursing and the medical director to be aware that spiritual intervention may need to run in parallel with any medication adjustment for this to actually work. Second, on Mrs. K.'s case, the family conflict over her code status is not primarily a medical disagreement. Her son and daughter are actually arguing a theological question underneath the DNR conversation — whether choosing comfort care equals giving up on faith that God can still heal her. I'd like to request a family meeting where I can be present specifically to address that theological tension directly, separate from the clinical conversation about prognosis. And third, on Mr. P.'s case, I'm recommending we increase his aide hours. His wife is his sole caregiver and she's showing clear signs of burnout — she broke down during my visit this week and told me she hasn't slept a full night in over two weeks. I don't think this is a spiritual care fix; I think this is a staffing and respite issue, and I wanted the full team to hear it from me directly rather than buried in a note."*

***Corresponding Chart Note (DAROP Format):***

**DATA:** This chaplain identifies a clinically significant pattern across three active cases warranting interdisciplinary attention. Mr. D. reports that existential and spiritual anxiety regarding death correlates directly with increased subjective pain reporting, independent of any change in his physical condition, and describes his current morphine regimen as feeling "less effective" during periods of heightened spiritual distress. Mrs. K.'s adult children are in ongoing conflict regarding her code status, which upon assessment is rooted in a theological disagreement about whether comfort care measures represent a loss of faith in God's healing power, rather than a purely medical disagreement about prognosis. Mr. P.'s wife, his sole caregiver, disclosed significant caregiver burnout during this chaplain's visit, including sleep deprivation exceeding two weeks and an emotional breakdown during the encounter.

**ACTION:** This chaplain presented all three findings verbally at IDG. For Mr. D., this chaplain recommended coordinated spiritual and medication intervention rather than medication adjustment alone. For Mrs. K., this chaplain requested and was granted authorization to facilitate a family meeting specifically addressing the theological dimension of the code status conflict, separate from the medical prognosis conversation. For Mr. P., this chaplain formally recommended increased aide hours to the team based on observed and disclosed caregiver burnout.

**RESULTS:** IDG concurred with all three recommendations. Medical director agreed to reassess Mr. D.'s pain management plan in coordination with this chaplain's continued spiritual care visits. Social work agreed to co-facilitate the family meeting for Mrs. K. with this chaplain. Case manager approved an increase in aide hours for Mr. P.'s household pending authorization review.

**OBSERVATIONS:** These three cases illustrate the clinical relevance of spiritual assessment data to pain management, family systems conflict, and caregiver capacity, respectively. Spiritual distress is not a parallel, separate concern from the medical plan of care in any of these cases; it is directly influencing clinical outcomes.

**PLAN:** This chaplain will follow up on Mr. D.'s pain and anxiety correlation at next week's visit and report back to the medical director. This chaplain will co-facilitate the family meeting for Mrs. K. within the next seven days. This chaplain will monitor Mr. P.'s wife's caregiver status following the aide hour increase and reassess in two weeks.

**Why This Works:** About as clear a demonstration as you'll find of why chaplains belong at the table and not just in the chart. The verbal report translates spiritual assessment into language the whole team can act on — pain management, family meeting logistics, staffing decisions — without losing the spiritual substance underneath each recommendation. The chart note preserves that same translation permanently, so the reasoning survives past the moment the meeting ends.

**CPE Learning Edge:** IDG reporting is a formation exercise in itself. It asks you to hold your spiritual assessment with enough confidence to say, out loud, in front of a room of clinicians, that a theological conflict is driving a code status disagreement, or spiritual anxiety is undermining pain control. New chaplains often soften a claim like that into vague language, afraid of overstepping into medical territory. Learning to speak your clinical spiritual assessment with the same clarity a nurse uses to report a change in vital signs is part of your growth as a chaplain, and part of what CPEI formation is specifically training you toward as a future supervisor.

**Patterns Across the Eight**

Before we move on, worth naming what these eight notes share, because the patterns matter more than any single example. In every one of them, the chaplain resisted at least one strong pull toward a lesser note. In Scenario A, the pull was toward manufacturing spiritual distress that wasn't there. In B, toward pathologizing a coping style that just looked different from the chaplain's own. In C, toward writing "resolved her distress" when nothing was resolved and nothing needed to be. In D, toward minimizing a passive death wish, or overreacting to it. In E, toward manufacturing evidence of a response the chaplain couldn't actually verify. In F, toward writing the chaplain's own emotional experience into a note that belonged to the family. In G, toward correcting a patient's spiritual disconnection instead of naming it honestly. In H, toward softening a clinical claim out of fear of overstepping.

Eight different pulls, eight chaplains resisting them, and underneath all eight is the same discipline: stay close to what actually happened, trust that the truth is more useful than the flattering version, and let your theology hold whatever you observe instead of needing the observation to already be resolved or comfortable. That discipline travels. It'll cover you in encounters this book never thought to include.

**FOR REFLECTION**

- *Which of these eight scenarios most resembles a visit already on your caseload this month? What would change in your own note if you borrowed its structure?*
- *Look back at Scenario D. Do you have a documented process for same-day RN notification and IDG presentation when a passive death wish surfaces? If not, who do you need to talk to this week?*
- *In Scenario H, the chaplain speaks with real clinical confidence about spiritual distress driving a medical outcome. Where in your own IDG participation do you soften your language more than the clinical picture warrants?*

# Chapter 6
# Six More Encounters — Expanding the Casebook

The eight scenarios in the last chapter cover a lot of ground, but no caseload stays inside those eight boundaries for long. This chapter adds six more, drawn from the wider range of situations hospice chaplains actually walk into — a dying child, a family whose faith tradition isn't your own, siblings in disagreement over their mother's care, a patient still actively using substances, a patient whose life you may not fully understand but are still called to serve without condition, and a moment of your own moral distress inside the interdisciplinary team.

I chose these six on purpose. Each one exposes a different kind of edge — theological, cultural, relational, ethical — and I've watched chaplains, including myself early on, get caught flat-footed by exactly these kinds of encounters more than by anything covered in a standard orientation. A caseload heavy on straightforward, same-culture, same-faith patients can lull a chaplain into believing their existing toolkit is enough. It rarely stays enough for long.

# Scenario I: Pediatric Hospice — Parents and Siblings — Memorial Hermann Five-Part Model

**Patient: Noah T., 6-year-old male, DIPG (diffuse intrinsic pontine glioma)**

**REASON FOR VISIT:** This chaplain visited at the request of the primary nurse following a difficult morning in which Noah's parents, Kayla and Marcus, received an updated prognosis indicating a significantly shortened life expectancy. Older sibling Ava, age 9, was present in the home during the visit.

**INTERVENTIONS:** This chaplain met first with Kayla and Marcus alone, allowing them space to voice raw anger and grief without needing to protect Ava from witnessing it. Kayla stated, "I have prayed every single day for a miracle, and I am starting to be angry at God for not giving me one." This chaplain did not rush to defend God or resolve her anger, instead naming that her anger is itself a form of relationship with God, not a rejection of Him. This chaplain then met briefly and separately with Ava, using developmentally appropriate, concrete language rather than euphemism, and invited her to draw a picture of anything she wanted her brother to know. Ava drew a picture of herself and Noah together and stated, "I want him to know I'm not mad he gets more attention." This chaplain gently normalized sibling feelings of resentment alongside love, without judgment.

**OUTCOMES:** Kayla wept during the conversation about her anger and stated she felt "less crazy" hearing that anger at God was not spiritually forbidden. Ava appeared visibly relieved after naming her mixed feelings and asked if she could keep her drawing to give to Noah.

**ASSESSMENT:** Family is entering acute anticipatory grief with theological distress centered on unanswered prayer for healing. Sibling Ava is at risk for disenfranchised grief given the family's necessary focus on Noah's care; her mixed feelings of love and resentment are developmentally normal and were appropriately validated rather than pathologized.

**PLAN:** This chaplain will continue weekly family visits, with separate, age-appropriate engagement for Ava at each visit. This chaplain will coordinate with the hospice's social worker regarding sibling support resources and will introduce the concept of a legacy project (recording, memory box) at the next visit, timed to the family's readiness rather than imposed on a schedule.

**Why This Works:** This note handles two patients at once, the dying child and the grieving-in-advance sibling, without collapsing their needs into one undifferentiated "family support" line. It also does something theologically important — it refuses to defend God against Kayla's anger, which is the anti-transactional move this book has argued for since Chapter One. Anger at God, held honestly, sits closer to biblical lament than a forced, premature peace would.

**CPE Learning Edge:** Pediatric hospice tests a chaplain's own theology of suffering harder than almost anything else, because no framework, not even a good one, makes a child's death make sense. Newer chaplains often feel pressure to have an answer for why, and the absence of a satisfying answer can trigger either theological retreat — silence, generic comfort — or theological overreach, offering explanations Scripture itself doesn't offer. Write down exactly what you said, and ask your supervisor honestly whether you offered Kayla presence or a theology you needed to believe more than she did.

# Scenario J: Interfaith Care — A Muslim Patient and Family — SOAP Format

**Patient: Mr. Hassan A., 74-year-old male, pancreatic cancer**

**SUBJECTIVE:** This chaplain, a Christian, was assigned to Mr. A.'s case following the family's request for "spiritual support," without a stated preference against a chaplain outside their Islamic tradition. Son Tariq, present as translator and primary decision-maker, stated, "My father wants to know someone is praying for him, but he wants his own imam for the important things." Mr. A., through his son, expressed concern about maintaining his daily prayers (salat) as his physical condition declines.

**OBJECTIVE:** Patient was alert, resting in a hospital bed positioned to allow him to face what the family identified as the direction of Mecca. A prayer rug was visible, folded near the bed. Patient's affect was calm; he nodded and made brief eye contact during the visit.

**ASSESSMENT:** Patient has an active, clear spiritual practice and support structure through his own faith community and does not require this chaplain to provide religious instruction or ritual leadership outside that tradition. Appropriate chaplain role in this case is respectful presence, practical support for maintaining religious practice, and coordination with the patient's own imam rather than substitution for that relationship.

**PLAN:** This chaplain will coordinate with nursing to ensure care activities are scheduled, where clinically possible, to avoid interrupting the patient's five daily prayer times, and will confirm with the family the best way to facilitate a visit from the patient's imam. This chaplain will continue brief supportive visits focused on presence rather than religious content, and will ask the family directly, at each visit, whether this chaplain's continued involvement remains welcome.

**Why This Works:** Something chaplains across every tradition need more practice doing: staying in your lane with humility while still being genuinely useful. The chaplain doesn't attempt to lead Islamic prayer or offer theological content outside their competence and calling. Instead the note documents concrete, practical support — prayer-time scheduling, imam coordination — that serves the patient's actual religious practice. It also documents an ongoing consent check, which matters a great deal in interfaith care. A family's welcome of a chaplain from outside their tradition can change. A good chaplain checks instead of assuming.

**CPE Learning Edge:** Interfaith encounters often surface a quiet anxiety in chaplains formed in a single tradition — am I even allowed to be useful here if I'm not the primary religious authority? The answer is yes, but the use of self that is required is different than in same-tradition care. You aren't the theological expert in the room, and that being present without being the expert is its own form of ministry. Bring to supervision any moment you felt the urge to over-explain your own faith instead of simply serving the patient's.

# Scenario K: Family Conflict Over Care Decisions — DAROP Format

**Patient: Mrs. Doris W., 89-year-old female, advanced dementia**

**DATA:** This chaplain was called by the case manager due to escalating conflict between Mrs. W.'s two adult daughters, Renee and Carla, regarding whether their mother should remain at Renee's home under hospice care or be transferred to a facility. Renee stated, "I promised her I'd never put her in a home, and Carla is trying to make me break that promise." Carla stated, "Renee is exhausted and won't admit it, and I'm scared Mom isn't getting safe care anymore." Both daughters became tearful during the conversation; no verbal or physical hostility observed during this chaplain's visit.

**ACTION:** This chaplain met with both daughters together, with their consent, and named directly that this conflict is not really about logistics — it is two daughters each trying, in different ways, to be faithful to their mother and to love her well. This chaplain did not take a position on the placement decision itself, which is outside this chaplain's clinical scope, and instead created space for each daughter to voice her fear underneath her position: Renee's fear of breaking a sacred promise, Carla's fear of her mother suffering unseen. This chaplain reflected both fears back to the room without ranking them.

**RESULTS:** Both daughters acknowledged, for the first time in this chaplain's presence, that the other was acting out of love rather than malice. Renee stated, "I didn't realize how scared you actually are." No resolution to the placement question was reached during this visit, nor was that the goal.

**OBSERVATIONS:** Family conflict is rooted in divergent expressions of loyalty and fear rather than disagreement about their mother's worth or their love for her. This is a family systems and care-planning issue requiring social work and case management involvement alongside ongoing spiritual support; it is not primarily a spiritual distress issue in the patient herself, who remains stable and comfortable per nursing report.

**PLAN:** This chaplain recommended a joint family meeting facilitated by the social worker and case manager to address the placement decision directly, with this chaplain available to attend in a supportive, non-directive role if the family requests it. This chaplain will follow up individually with Renee, given her role as primary caregiver, to assess her own caregiver burden separately from the family conflict.

**Why This Works:** A clean, important line. The chaplain names the emotional and spiritual dynamics driving the conflict without wading into the clinical or logistical decision itself. That restraint isn't passivity. It's precise role clarity, and it's exactly what lets the chaplain be trusted by both daughters instead of perceived as taking a side.

**CPE Learning Edge:** Family conflict visits pull hard at the fixer instinct, because there's an actual decision that needs making and every fiber of your training might want to help make it. The task here is distinguishing between facilitating emotional honesty, which is squarely chaplaincy's job, and adjudicating a care decision, which is not. Notice yourself forming an opinion about which daughter is right? That opinion belongs in supervision. Not in the room, not in the chart.

# Scenario L: Spiritual Care Amid Active Substance Use — Spiritual AIM Format

**Patient: Mr. Tyrell J., 54-year-old male, end-stage renal disease**

**ASSESSMENT (Domain:** Self-Worth): Patient disclosed ongoing use of alcohol and, per his report, occasional marijuana use for pain and nausea management, describing significant shame around both his diagnosis and his substance use history. Patient stated, "I know what people think when they hear 'still using.' They think I don't want to get better. I just want to not hurt for a few hours." This chaplain assessed a deeply held belief that his worth is contingent on sobriety he has been unable to sustain, and that this belief is a primary barrier to him accepting spiritual or emotional support of any kind.

**INTERVENTION:** This chaplain explicitly separated the clinical and harm-reduction conversation, which remains the medical team's domain, from the spiritual conversation, which is this chaplain's domain, and named directly that God's love for him was never contingent on his sobriety in the first place. This chaplain did not challenge, minimize, or moralize about his substance use, and instead reflected that his shame, not his use itself, appeared to be the heavier burden he was carrying into this conversation.

**OUTCOME (Domain:** Self-Worth): Patient's shoulders visibly relaxed and he stated, "Nobody's ever said it like that to me before, that God's not waiting on me to get clean." Patient agreed to continued visits and, unprompted, asked this chaplain to pray with him before the visit ended, which had not occurred in prior visits.

**PLAN:** This chaplain will continue weekly visits with continued focus on unconditional worth rather than behavioral change, which remains outside this chaplain's clinical role. This chaplain will coordinate with nursing regarding any harm-reduction resources appropriate to his goals of care, and will monitor for any shift toward readiness for deeper spiritual or reconciliation work as trust builds.

**Why This Works:** A direct, practical application of the anti-transactional theology from Chapter Three — you are loved before you perform. It also models a real boundary. The chaplain doesn't become an amateur addiction counselor and doesn't use the visit to advocate for sobriety, which isn't the chaplain's lane and would have undermined the actual spiritual work available in that room.

**CPE Learning Edge:** Patients with active substance use often carry an accurate prediction that religious or spiritual caregivers will moralize at them, because many have experienced exactly that from churches or well-meaning family. The learning edge here is noticing your own reflexive judgment before it reaches your face, your tone, or your note. If your documentation of a patient like this one contains language that reads as disapproval rather than clinical observation, that's worth examining with your supervisor. Not because you're a bad chaplain for having the reaction. Because an unexamined reaction like that eventually leaks into the room.

# Scenario M: Presence Without Condition — DAROP Format

**Patient: Ms. Diane P., 61-year-old female, ovarian cancer, partnered with Ms. Karen L.**

**DATA:** This chaplain visited at patient's request for "someone to talk to about dying." Patient's partner of eighteen years, Karen, was present. Patient disclosed she was raised in a conservative religious household that she left in her twenties, stating, "I left my church a long time ago because I didn't think there was room for me there. I don't know if I believe in much of anything anymore, but I don't want to die without talking to somebody about it." Patient did not request denominational or doctrinal guidance and did not ask this chaplain's personal theological views.

**ACTION:** This chaplain listened to patient's spiritual history without correcting, defending, or relitigating the tradition she left, and affirmed that her presence in this conversation — showing up honestly, uncertain and searching — is itself a legitimate spiritual posture. This chaplain asked what, if anything, still felt sacred to her, and patient identified her relationship with Karen and the eighteen years they have built together as "the realest, most sacred thing in my life." This chaplain reflected that back without qualification. At patient's request, this chaplain offered a closing prayer using open, inclusive language focused on comfort, presence, and Karen, rather than theology the patient had not requested.

**RESULTS:** Patient became tearful and stated, "That's the first time a chaplain didn't make me feel like I had to explain myself." Karen thanked this chaplain audibly at the end of the visit. Patient agreed to further visits.

**OBSERVATIONS:** Patient presents with spiritual openness and genuine searching following past religious wounding. Primary spiritual need at this time is unconditional presence and freedom from anticipated judgment, not doctrinal instruction. Relationship with Karen functions as patient's primary source of meaning and sacred connection.

**PLAN:** This chaplain will continue visits focused on presence and open listening, following patient's lead regarding any spiritual or religious content she wishes to explore. This chaplain will include Karen in visits per patient's preference and will monitor for any expressed desire for more specific religious engagement, which will be honored if and when patient initiates it.

**Why This Works:** A model of hospice chaplaincy's foundational ethical commitment is serving the spiritual needs of every patient as that patient defines them, without imposing the chaplain's own theological framework. Diane didn't ask for doctrine. She asked for presence. The chaplain gave her exactly what was asked for, and the note documents that restraint as a clinical choice, not an absence of conviction.

**CPE Learning Edge:** Every chaplain carries personal theological convictions into every room, mine included, and I've been honest about that throughout this book. The formation task in this scenario isn't pretending you have no convictions. It's holding them with enough discipline that a patient who's been hurt by religious judgment before doesn't encounter that judgment from you, even silently, even in your face. If you find you can't offer a patient like Diane unconditional presence without your own theology intruding, that's exactly the kind of use-of-self material a verbatim and a trusted supervisor exist to help you work through. The APC Standards of Practice are explicit that chaplains serve the spiritual needs of the patient as the patient defines them. Our role is presence. Not persuasion.

# Scenario N: Moral Distress and IDG Conflict — Memorial Hermann Five-Part Model

**Context: Team conflict regarding Mr. Owens, 82-year-old male, end-stage COPD**

**REASON FOR VISIT/ENTRY:** This chaplain is documenting a moment of professional disagreement at IDG regarding Mr. Owens's care, in keeping with agency policy that significant team conflicts affecting patient care be reflected in the record. Mr. Owens has repeatedly and consistently stated a wish to remain at home and decline further hospitalization. His son, who holds medical power of attorney, has requested an aggressive readmission for a treatable infection, against the patient's previously expressed wishes and current capacity to communicate those wishes himself.

**INTERVENTIONS:** This chaplain advocated at IDG for honoring Mr. Owens's directly and repeatedly stated wishes, noting that when he was cognitively intact he was unambiguous in multiple documented conversations, including with this chaplain, that he does not want further hospitalization. This chaplain recommended an ethics consultation given the disagreement between the medical POA holder and the patient's own voice.

**OUTCOMES:** The team agreed to convene an ethics consultation prior to any transfer decision and to conduct a direct capacity assessment with Mr. Owens. This chaplain's advocacy was received respectfully by the team, though this chaplain notes ongoing internal moral distress regarding the possibility that the patient's voice may still be overridden.

**ASSESSMENT:** This is a case of significant ethical complexity involving surrogate decision-making authority in tension with a previously competent patient's expressed wishes. This chaplain's role is to ensure the patient's voice remains centered in the team's decision-making process, not to guarantee a particular outcome, which is outside any single team member's control.

**PLAN:** This chaplain will continue supporting Mr. Owens directly, will attend the ethics consultation as the patient's spiritual care provider, and will process this chaplain's own moral distress in individual supervision this week, separate from the clinical documentation of the case.

**Why This Works:** Something rarely modeled in chaplaincy training — how to document your own professional advocacy and disagreement inside a team, clinically, without editorializing about colleagues. It also does something for the field's credibility. It shows a chaplain functioning as an ethical voice at the table, not merely a source of comfort, which is exactly the expanded role our profession is being asked to fill.

**CPE Learning Edge:** This scenario names something CPE formation doesn't always address directly enough: chaplains experience genuine moral distress, and that distress needs its own container. Notice the last line of the note — this chaplain will process moral distress in individual supervision, separate from the clinical documentation. That's not filler. It's a boundary protecting both the chart's clinical integrity and the chaplain's own wellbeing. A chaplain who never names their own moral distress to a supervisor is accumulating exactly the kind of unprocessed weight that leads to the burnout described in Chapter One. Don't let that happen to you. Bring it to supervision. Every time.

**Patterns Across the Six**

These six stretch further than the original eight on purpose, because a career in hospice chaplaincy will eventually stretch you further than your training prepared you for. Notice how the chaplain's clinical role stays remarkably consistent even as the content varies wildly — a dying child, a patient of another faith, a family feud, a patient still using substances, a patient whose life the chaplain may not have shared every conviction about, a colleague-facing ethical conflict. In every case the chaplain's job was not having the perfect theological answer. It was staying present, staying honest about what was and wasn't within their scope, and documenting with enough precision that whoever touches the case next understands exactly what happened and why.

One more thread runs through all six. Every single scenario asked the chaplain to hold a tension rather than resolve it. Kayla's anger at God wasn't resolved. Mr. A.'s family's need for their own imam alongside a hospice chaplain wasn't resolved into a single relationship. Renee and Carla's disagreement about their mother's placement wasn't resolved by the chaplain, and wasn't supposed to be. Mr. Owens's ethical situation wasn't resolved by the chaplain's advocacy alone. Hospice chaplaincy, done honestly, spends far more time holding unresolved tension well than it spends producing tidy resolutions. If you came into this work hoping to be the one who fixes things, I hope by now you're starting to feel the relief of setting that hope down. Witnessing well, tension and all, is enough. It was always enough.

**FOR REFLECTION**

- *Of these six, which one sits furthest outside your comfort zone, and what makes it uncomfortable — a gap in training, a gap in theology, or a gap in personal experience?*
- *Scenario M asks a chaplain to offer unconditional presence to a patient whose life experience may differ from the chaplain's own convictions. Where is your own edge on that kind of encounter, and who do you talk to when you reach it?*
- *Do you have a real, reliable place to process your own moral distress? Not theoretically — a specific person, a specific rhythm. If not, what's one step you could take this month?*

# Chapter 7
# CPE and the Charting Life — Verbatims, Supervision, and Self-Reflection

If you came up through Clinical Pastoral Education, you already own the core discipline good charting requires. You may just not have connected the two yet. This chapter makes that connection explicit, because it may be the single most useful reframe I can offer a chaplain who sat through at least one unit of CPE and assumed the verbatim process was something you left behind once you got certified.

A verbatim, for anyone reading this who hasn't done CPE, is a written reconstruction of a pastoral encounter (as close to word-for-word as memory allows) followed by theological and psychological reflection on what happened in the room, in the patient, and in the chaplain.

A good verbatim has a recognizable shape: a brief description of the setting and the patient, a dialogue reconstruction that honestly tries to capture what was actually said rather than an idealized version of the conversation, and then a reflection section where the chaplain names what they noticed about their own internal reactions, their theological assumptions, and the countertransference at play. That reflection section is where the real formation happens. It's where a peer group and a supervisor see not just what you did, but why, and whether the why holds up under examination.

The verbatim process trains you to do three things in sequence.

*Observe carefully.*

*Record what actually happened rather than what you wish had happened or remember happening.*

*Then analyze that record for what it reveals about the patient, the dynamics in the room, and yourself.*

That is almost exactly what a good chart note requires. A chaplain who has done real verbatim work, who has sat with a peer group and had someone point out that the dialogue they wrote doesn't quite match what they described feeling in the room, has already built the muscle for honest documentation. The daily chart note is the verbatim discipline applied at a much smaller scale, many times a week, without a peer group to catch your blind spots. Which is exactly why the discipline matters more in daily practice, not less. Nobody is checking your work the way your CPE group did.

Imagine a verbatim excerpt like this:

> *"I asked the patient how she was feeling about her diagnosis. She said, 'I don't know, I guess I'm okay.' I told her that it was normal to feel scared, and that God has a plan for her even in this. She nodded and looked out the window. I said a prayer and left."*

Any CPE supervisor worth their credential stops a student cold on that verbatim, because it's full of exactly the moves this book has spent six chapters training you out of. The chaplain told the patient what she should be feeling — scared — rather than asking. The chaplain offered a theological claim, God has a plan, that the patient never requested and that may not have landed the way the chaplain intended. She "looked out the window" rather than responding, and that's data the chaplain never processed. The chaplain closed the encounter with a prayer and an exit rather than staying with the patient's actual, ambiguous "I guess I'm okay."

Now watch what happens when that same chaplain, having done the reflective work a verbatim demands, charts the visit honestly instead of charitably. A witness's version might read:

> *"Patient stated, 'I don't know, I guess I'm okay,' regarding her diagnosis. When this chaplain offered reassurance, patient did not verbally respond and turned to look out the window; this chaplain did not further explore this nonverbal cue during the visit. Plan: this chaplain will use more open-ended questioning at next visit and will directly explore patient's response to the window moment, given the ambiguity of her nonverbal reaction."*

Not a flattering note. It documents a missed opportunity honestly, and that honesty is exactly what makes it useful — to the chaplain's own growth, to a supervisor reviewing the case, and to the next chaplain who might pick up this chart and know to slow down and ask about that window.

**From Fixer to Witness**

This brings us to the learning edge every CPE student wrestles with in some form, whether their supervisor has named it explicitly or not: the shift from fixer to witness. Most of us came into chaplaincy from some prior life — ministry, counseling, teaching — where our value was measured by whether we solved the problem in front of us. CPE formation exists in large part to dismantle that reflex, because a fixer at a deathbed isn't just unhelpful. It can be actively harmful, foreclosing exactly the space a dying person needs to have their own experience rather than manage the chaplain's need to be useful. This shift shows up in your documentation in specific, checkable ways.

- A fixer's note is heavy on interpretation and light on observation — "patient is in denial," "family is dysfunctional," "patient needs to accept reality" — conclusions dressed up as assessments, built on the chaplain's own theory of what should be happening rather than what was actually witnessed.
- A witness's note reverses that ratio. It stays close to specific, observable data — what was said, what was seen, what changed — and holds interpretation more lightly, offering it as clinical reasoning rather than verdict.
- A fixer's note is heavy on advice given. A witness's note is heavy on presence offered and space held.
- A fixer's note, read closely, is often subtly performing competence for whoever reads it next. A witness's note is simply available, unadorned, and accurate.

Go back through your last ten notes with this lens and you'll learn something real about where you currently sit on that spectrum. This isn't a spectrum any of us graduate from permanently, and I'll say honestly that I still catch fixer language in my own drafts more often than I'd like, especially on days when I'm tired and reaching for the note that will let me close the chart fastest. The goal isn't never slipping. It's developing the internal alarm that notices the slip before the note is finalized.

### Countertransference and the Chart

Now the harder conversation: countertransference and the chart. Every chaplain eventually meets a patient who reminds them, uncomfortably, of their own family, their own unresolved grief, their own trauma. That's an inevitable consequence of doing this work as an actual human being rather than a detached technician. The danger isn't that countertransference happens. The danger is that it happens invisibly and finds its way into the chart disguised as clinical observation.

If a patient's estrangement from his children echoes your own family history, you're at real risk of writing a note that subtly editorializes his situation through your own unprocessed feelings about yours — overstating his guilt, or understating it, or projecting a resolution onto the relationship that you wish existed in your own life. A second illustration helps, because this pattern is easier to describe abstractly than catch in yourself. Suppose a chaplain whose own mother died after a long, isolating illness is assigned to a patient whose adult daughter visits infrequently. A countertransference-driven note might read, "*Daughter appears emotionally distant and minimally engaged in patient's care,*" when the observable facts are simply that the daughter lives four hours away and works full time. The chaplain's own grief about a mother who felt abandoned has quietly reshaped "*distance*" into "*distant*" — a factual observation into a character judgment. The safeguard here isn't willpower. It's supervision. When you notice a visit has stirred something in you disproportionate to what actually happened in the room, that's data for your next supervision session or peer group, not raw material for the chart. Write what you observed in the patient. Bring what you felt in yourself to the people whose job it is to help you metabolize it. Keeping those two streams separate, consistently, is one of the clearest signs of a chaplain who has done real formation work.

# A Self-Assessment Exercise

**A Self-Assessment Exercise**

Here's a brief exercise I'd ask every chaplain reading this book to actually do, not just read about. If you're working through this book with a CPE cohort or a staff training group, it translates well into a peer-group session — have each chaplain bring one note, read it aloud with names redacted, and let the group ask the four questions together. Done in community, this exercise recovers some of what a lone chaplain loses without a verbatim peer group.

Pull your last ten chart notes. For each one, ask four questions.

1. Did I include at least one direct patient quote, in their own words?
2. Did I record a specific, observable outcome, not just "patient appeared to benefit"?
3. Would another chaplain, reading only this note, understand exactly what I did and why I chose to do it?
4. Is there any sentence in this note that says more about me than it does about the patient?

Answer those four questions honestly across ten notes and you'll know where your documentation needs to grow. That's a far better teacher than a vague sense that your charting "should probably be better."

# A Full Verbatim, Start to Finish

It helps to see one complete verbatim, in something closer to its full CPE form, so every piece of the process we've been discussing lands together. What follows is a composite, built to illustrate the form rather than describe an actual encounter.

*Setting: Home visit, hospice patient, 79-year-old male, prostate cancer, week two of service. Present: patient, this chaplain. Patient was seated in a recliner, oxygen off, alert.*

*Reflection: My urge at C3-C4 to reassure him that "it will work out" is worth naming honestly. I think it came from my own discomfort with unresolved father-son material — my relationship with my own father has threads I haven't fully worked through, and I noticed myself wanting to resolve his situation partly to avoid sitting with mine. I'm glad I caught the urge before I spoke it, and I want to bring this specific reaction to supervision, because I suspect it will recur with other patients whose family estrangements echo shapes in my own history. Theologically, what this patient needed most today was permission not to know yet whether forgiveness or an apology comes first — an anti-transactional, non-resolving kind of presence — rather than a chaplain rushing him toward either.*

Now watch how that verbatim translates into a chart note, using DAROP format. Notice what carries over and what doesn't.

**DATA:** Patient alert, seated in recliner, oxygen off. Patient disclosed his estranged adult son visited the previous day for the first time in six years. Patient stated, "I don't know yet if I'm supposed to forgive him or if he's supposed to be asking me to."

**ACTION:** This chaplain offered open-ended reflection rather than premature reassurance, naming that the patient appeared uncertain which direction reconciliation needed to move. This chaplain offered prayer, which patient declined in favor of continued silence; this chaplain remained present in silence per patient's preference for several additional minutes.

**RESULTS:** Patient confirmed the chaplain's reflection ("Yeah, that's it exactly") and appeared to settle into the silence rather than continuing to search for resolution during this visit.

**OBSERVATIONS:** Patient is in the early stages of processing an unexpected reconciliation opportunity with an estranged son after six years of separation. Patient does not yet have clarity about the shape reconciliation should take and appears to need space to sit with that ambiguity rather than pressure to resolve it quickly.

**PLAN:** This chaplain will follow up specifically on the son relationship at next visit, without pressing for resolution, and will monitor for patient's readiness to explore next steps, including a possible facilitated conversation with the son if patient expresses interest.

Notice what didn't make it into the chart note: the chaplain's own countertransference regarding their father. Real, and it mattered, but it belonged entirely in the reflection section of the verbatim and in supervision, not in the patient's medical record. That's the whole discipline of this chapter in miniature. The verbatim can hold everything, because it's a formation document written for you and your supervisor. The chart note holds only what serves the patient's ongoing care, written for the whole team. Knowing which material belongs in which document is itself a clinical skill worth practicing deliberately.

**Building a Peer Group Where None Exists**

Most staff chaplains, once they leave a CPE program, lose access to the single structure that made their formation possible: a regular peer group with a trained supervisor holding the room. That's a real loss, and our field doesn't talk about it honestly enough. Charting alone, without any peer accountability, is harder to sustain at a high standard indefinitely — not because you lack discipline, but because none of us can see our own blind spots without another set of eyes.

If your hospice doesn't have a formal chaplain peer review structure, build one, even informally, even small. It doesn't need to be a full verbatim group meeting weekly. It can be two chaplains agreeing to trade one redacted chart note a month and ask each other the four self-assessment questions from this chapter, out loud, honestly. It can be a monthly seminar, like the one this book grew out of, where a team gathers to workshop real charting challenges together. The format matters less than the fact that your writing gets seen by another set of trained eyes on some kind of regular rhythm — because the alternative, writing in permanent isolation, accountable only to yourself, is exactly the condition under which fixer language, countertransference, and quiet burnout all creep in unnoticed. I built the monthly seminar structure that produced this book, in large part, because I needed that accountability for myself as much as I needed to offer it to the chaplains I supervise.

# A Note to Supervisors and Supervisors-in-Training

### A Note to Supervisors and Supervisors-in-Training

I'm writing this book, in part, while sitting inside my own CPEI training, being formed as someone who will eventually supervise other chaplains through exactly the process just described. A word directly to anyone reading this who supervises chaplains or is preparing to: the temptation, when reviewing a student's or a staff chaplain's notes, is to focus entirely on format compliance — did they use the right acronym, did they fill in every field.

Format compliance matters, but it's the smallest part of what a good documentation review should accomplish. The deeper question, every time, is the same one this chapter has been building toward. ***Does this note observe, or does it interpret prematurely? Does it witness, or does it perform?*** Teaching a chaplain to answer that honestly about their own writing is one of the most transferable formation skills a supervisor can offer, because a chaplain who can see the fixer creeping into their chart note can usually see it creeping into the room too, before it does damage.

One more before-and-after, because a second example makes the pattern stick better than a single one ever could. Imagine a verbatim excerpt where a chaplain writes: "The patient's daughter was very difficult and kept interrupting our conversation with questions about medication. I finally had to ask her to let me finish talking with her father." Read that closely. Every clause carries a judgment — very difficult, interrupting, finally had to ask. None of it tells us what the daughter actually said, or what her questions actually were, or what might have been driving her need to ask them in the first place. A witness's version, written after real reflection, might read instead: "Patient's daughter asked three questions during the visit regarding her father's current pain medication dosage. This chaplain paused the spiritual conversation to acknowledge her questions were important and suggested she raise them with the nurse after this visit, then resumed conversation with the patient." Same event. Completely different note. The second version lets a reader form their own judgment about the daughter's behavior, probably a far more generous one than "very difficult," because it gives them the actual facts instead of the chaplain's interpretation of those facts. That's the entire discipline of this chapter, distilled into two sentences: give the reader the facts, and trust them, and yourself, with the interpretation.

## FOR REFLECTION

- *Pull one recent chart note and try the verbatim treatment on it: rewrite the encounter as if reconstructing dialogue for a peer group. What does that slower, more honest reconstruction reveal that your original note missed?*
- *Name a specific patient who has stirred countertransference in you recently. What is the observable fact you may have quietly reshaped into a judgment, and where does that feeling actually belong?*
- *If you supervise or mentor other chaplains, how much of your documentation feedback currently focuses on format versus the deeper question of witness versus performance? What would it look like to rebalance that?*

# Chapter 8
# Regulatory, Legal, and Ethical Guardrails

This chapter is devoted entirely to the plain regulatory and legal realities sitting underneath everything said so far. Pastoral integrity and regulatory compliance aren't in tension here. They point in the same direction, and chaplains are better served understanding the why behind these requirements than experiencing them as arbitrary hoops.

**The Conditions of Participation**

The Medicare Conditions of Participation require an initial spiritual assessment within five days of the election of the hospice benefit, and ongoing spiritual care documented as part of the plan of care throughout the length of stay, not just at admission. If your chart shows a spiritual assessment on day one and then silence for the next six weeks, you've created a regulatory gap regardless of how much actual spiritual care occurred in the room. The chart is the only evidence of care that exists once the visit is over, which brings us back to the theology of Chapter Three: if it isn't written, in the eyes of the regulation, it didn't happen.

Some texture here that a purely regulatory summary tends to miss.

The Conditions of Participation frame spiritual care as an interdisciplinary responsibility, not a chaplain's private domain. This means that the hospice team as a whole is required to address spiritual needs identified in the comprehensive assessment. That's actually good news for chaplains who sometimes feel isolated on their team, carrying the "spiritual box" alone. Regulatorily speaking, spiritual care is supposed to be everyone's job, coordinated through you as the specialist, which is one more reason your documentation needs to be legible and useful to non-chaplains. A note only you can interpret is a note that fails the interdisciplinary mandate baked into the regulation itself.

**Joint Commission Tracers**

Joint Commission tracer methodology, mentioned earlier, follows a single patient's record and asks whether an identified need led to a documented plan, and whether that plan was actually carried out over time. A beautifully written initial assessment that identifies a real spiritual need, followed by generic, interchangeable follow-up notes that never reference that need again, fails a tracer even though the initial documentation looked strong. Your plan needs to show up again in your outcomes, visit after visit, in a way a surveyor can literally trace. I've sat in more than one survey debrief where a chaplain's documentation was the single weakest link in an otherwise strong interdisciplinary chart, not because the care was poor, but because the paper trail didn't show the follow-through that had, in fact, happened at the bedside. Don't let good care go undocumented into a survey finding against your team.

**The APC Standard and the Word "Relevant"**

The Association of Professional Chaplains' standard puts the obligation simply: the chaplain documents, in the appropriate recording structure, information relevant to the care recipient's wellbeing. That word "relevant" is doing real work in that sentence. It's a standard against both extremes — the chaplain who writes nothing, and the chaplain who writes everything, including details that serve no one's understanding of the patient's spiritual condition and plan of care. I've reviewed notes on both ends of that spectrum. The empty note is the more common failure in my experience, but the overstuffed note — three paragraphs of theological reflection with no clear intervention or plan buried inside it — creates its own problem, because it buries the clinically actionable information a busy nurse or physician needs to find quickly. Relevant means enough, and not more than enough.

**HIPAA Basics for Chaplains**

I'm not an attorney, and nothing in this book should be taken as legal advice — for a specific situation, always consult your agency's compliance officer or legal counsel. But every chaplain should understand a few basic HIPAA principles well enough to apply them without looking them up under pressure.

- First: spiritual and religious information you gather as part of your clinical role is part of the medical record and is protected health information, just like a lab value or a medication list. It isn't somehow "more private" than clinical data in a way that exempts it from appropriate documentation, though it's subject to the same minimum-necessary standard as everything else — document what's clinically relevant to the plan of care, not every detail of a person's inner life.
- Second: sharing information within your interdisciplinary team for treatment purposes is fully permitted under HIPAA's treatment exception. The anxiety some chaplains feel about "breaking confidentiality" by charting for the IDG is, in almost every case, misplaced. The team is allowed to know what you know, when it serves the patient's care.
- Third: sharing information outside the treatment team, with a patient's home church, say, or a family member not involved in the care plan, requires the patient's

authorization, the same as it would for any other discipline. Confidentiality in chaplaincy isn't a separate, stricter standard than the rest of the medical record. It's the same standard, applied thoughtfully to spiritual and religious content.

### Confidentiality and Hearsay

Confidentiality and hearsay deserve their own careful attention, because chaplains hear things other disciplines don't, and the temptation to relay all of it uncritically into the chart is real. Document what you personally observed and what the patient personally told you, in their own words. Cite your source explicitly for any biomedical information you didn't personally witness — "per RN report" or "per chart review" — rather than presenting secondhand clinical information as your own direct observation. And be exact about the difference between a patient's self-disclosure and a family member's characterization of that patient. Never write *"per family, patient was a drunk."* Write instead, *"Patient stated he has struggled with alcohol use in the past."* The second version is both more accurate and more dignifying, and it happens to also be the version that holds up if this chart is ever read in a legal proceeding.

### Documentation as Quality Assurance

One more practical dimension worth naming: your notes aren't just a legal and clinical record. They're raw material for your agency's Quality Assessment and Performance Improvement program, which the Conditions of Participation require every hospice to maintain. QAPI committees look for patterns across charts — are spiritual needs identified at intake showing up addressed in the plan of care over time, are bereavement risk levels being reassessed at appropriate intervals, are high-risk safety disclosures like passive death wishes reliably reaching the IDG. A chaplaincy department with strong, consistent documentation gives its own QAPI committee real data to work with, which in turn gives your department a stronger voice in demonstrating its value to agency leadership. A chaplaincy department with thin, inconsistent documentation is, whether anyone says so out loud, effectively invisible to the quality improvement process. And departments invisible to quality improvement processes are, over time, the first departments cut when hospice margins tighten. I don't say that to frighten you into compliance. I say it because our profession needs to be able to demonstrate its own value in the same data-driven language the rest of healthcare increasingly requires, and good documentation is how we do that.

### Board Certification and the Standard You Are Held To

One more piece of the regulatory picture deserves a direct word: your board certification, or path toward it, sets a documentation standard even where your state doesn't license chaplains the way it licenses nurses or social workers.

Most states don't currently require a chaplaincy license to practice, which sometimes leads chaplains to conclude that documentation standards are, therefore, informal or optional. They aren't. Board Certified Chaplain status through bodies like the Association of Professional Chaplains carries its own Code of Ethics and Standards of Practice, and increasingly, hospice accrediting bodies and state hospice licensure surveys reference those standards directly when evaluating chaplain performance, certified or not.

If you're pursuing board certification, or supervising chaplains who are, treat the documentation standards in this book as inseparable from that credentialing process, not a separate compliance track running alongside it. The habits are the same habits either way.

**The Subpoena Reality**

Which brings us to the reality none of us likes to think about but all of us should write toward: the subpoena reality. Hospice charts get subpoenaed. Malpractice cases, disputed wills, guardianship disputes, and family conflicts over end-of-life decisions can all pull a chaplain's notes into a courtroom years after the visit itself is a distant memory to you. A composite illustration makes this concrete, built from patterns I've seen play out more than once across a career, though no single detail here describes an actual case. An adult child contests a parent's will two years after death, alleging the parent lacked capacity when a late-stage estate change was made. The hospice chart from that period becomes evidence. A chaplain's note from six weeks before death, stating simply "patient alert, oriented, engaged in meaningful conversation about family legacy," becomes a meaningful data point in a capacity argument neither the chaplain nor anyone else anticipated at the time. That isn't a reason to write differently than you otherwise would. It's a reason to write with the same specific, observed accuracy every single time, because you can't know in advance which ordinary Tuesday note will matter enormously two years later.

A word of reassurance closes this chapter, because a chapter full of regulations, tracers, HIPAA, and subpoenas can leave a pastoral heart feeling like the sacred work we started this book describing has quietly been replaced by a legal one. It hasn't. Every guardrail in this chapter exists in service of the same conviction running through every chapter before it: our patients and their families deserve a record faithful enough to be trusted, by anyone, at any time, for any reason. A regulator wants that record to prove the system worked. A grieving family wants that record to prove their loved one was truly seen. An attorney, in the rare case it comes to that, wants that record to establish what actually happened. All three audiences are, in the end, asking the same question a good chaplain should already be asking of every note they write: is this true, is this specific, and does it honor the person it describes? Meet that standard consistently, and every guardrail in this chapter takes care of itself.

Writing every note as though it might one day be read in a deposition isn't paranoia. It's simply writing with the level of care and precision our patients and their families deserve regardless of who else eventually reads it. A note built on direct observation, direct quotation, and honest clinical reasoning will always hold up, because it's simply true. That's the whole secret. There's no separate "legally defensible" writing style to learn. Accurate, specific, non-editorializing documentation is legally defensible documentation, because it's accurate.

**FOR REFLECTION**

- *Pull a chart from a patient still on your caseload. If a surveyor traced this chart tomorrow, would the plan you documented on day one still be visible in your most recent note?*
- *Think of a note you have written that contains secondhand information. Did you cite the source explicitly, or did it read as your own direct observation? What would you change about it now?*
- *Imagine your last five notes read aloud in a deposition two years from now. Which one would you be least comfortable having read back to you, and why?*

# Chapter 9
# Quick Reference Tools

This chapter is meant to be used, not just read. Photocopy it, tape it inside your work bag, or transcribe it into whatever quick-reference system your agency uses. These are the tools I hand every new chaplain I train, and the tools I still, after all these years, keep close enough to check myself against.

**The Charting Checklist — Run Through This for Every Note**

- Did I include at least one sensory or behavioral observation (affect, posture, breathing pattern, environment)?
- Did I include a direct quote from the patient or family member in their own words, wherever possible?
- Did I clearly name my intervention, not just the fact that I visited?
- Did I document the patient's or family's response to that intervention specifically, rather than a generic "patient was receptive"?
- Did I write a plan that includes a stated frequency, not just "continue to follow"?
- Would a chaplain who has never met this patient understand, from this note alone, exactly where they are on their spiritual journey right now?

A word on how to actually use this checklist. I've watched well-intentioned chaplains turn it into one more source of guilt rather than a genuine tool. You won't hit all six items on every single note, and that's fine — a two-minute PRN visit doesn't carry the same documentation weight as a comprehensive initial assessment. The checklist is a diagnostic, not a pass-fail test. If you consistently miss the same one or two items across many notes, that's useful information about a specific habit worth building. If you occasionally miss an item on a genuinely brief encounter, that's simply an accurate reflection of a brief encounter.

### Phrases That Help and Phrases That Hurt

- Replace "Patient was noncompliant" with "Patient declined the offered intervention."
- Replace "Manipulative family" with "Family expressed distress through repeated requests for information and updates."
- Replace "Patient is in denial" with "Patient states he is not currently ready to discuss prognosis."
- Replace "Difficult family dynamics" with a specific, observed description of the actual disagreement or behavior.
- Replace "Provided emotional support" with the specific thing you actually did — validated, listened, prayed, sat in silence, offered a specific reframe.
- Replace "Patient seemed at peace" with the specific behavioral or verbal evidence that led you to that clinical impression.

In every case the correction moves you from a vague, evaluative label toward a specific, observable description. That single habit will do more for your documentation than any framework in this book.

### Building Your Own Phrase Bank

The phrases-that-help list above is a starting point, not a finished vocabulary. Keep a running, personal phrase bank — a private document where you collect language that has worked well, specific and observable, whenever you write or read a note that hits the mark. Over a career, this becomes one of the most valuable documents you own, because it captures your own clinical voice at its best and gives you somewhere to reach on the days when your own words aren't coming easily. When I'm tired and reaching for a shortcut, I'd rather reach for a phrase I know is specific and honest than invent a vague one under deadline pressure. Build the bank now, before you need it on a hard day.

# How to Run a Fifteen-Minute Documentation Audit

Once a month, on a slow afternoon, run this audit on your own caseload. It takes about fifteen minutes and it'll tell you more about your documentation habits than any policy manual.

1. Pull five recent notes from five different patients, chosen quickly and at random rather than cherry-picked.
2. For each note, run the six-item Charting Checklist above and mark how many items it hits.
3. Read all five notes back to back, out loud if you can. Listen for repeated phrases, the same three or four sentences you reach for on autopilot across different patients. Circle any phrase that shows up more than twice.
4. Ask whether a stranger could tell these five patients apart from the notes alone, without the names attached. If the notes are interchangeable, that's your single most important finding.
5. Pick one specific habit to adjust for the next thirty days, not five habits, one, and revisit this audit next month to see whether it stuck.

I've run a version of this audit on my own charting for years, and I'll tell you honestly: it never stops being humbling, and it never stops being useful. The goal isn't catching yourself failing. It's keeping your writing honest enough that it could still surprise you, which is a good proxy for whether it's still specific enough to be worth reading.

# How to Run a Fifteen-Minute Documentation Audit

# 30-60-90 Day Documentation Onboarding Plan

### A 30-60-90 Day Documentation Onboarding Plan

If you're a hospice leader or CPE supervisor bringing a new chaplain onto your team, documentation formation deserves its own deliberate timeline, not a single orientation-day mention buried between benefits enrollment and badge photos. Here's the structure I use, adaptable to whatever framework your agency has chosen.

***Days 1-30: Observation and Foundation***

In the first thirty days, a new chaplain should read more notes than they write. Have them pull ten strong notes from your best documenters, redacted if needed, and walk through the Charting Checklist against each one together. Pair every new chaplain with a mentor who reviews their first two weeks of notes line by line, not as punishment but as active coaching, the same way a new nurse's first medication passes get double-checked. Introduce your agency's chosen documentation model in week one, and don't introduce a second model or a set of exceptions until the first one is genuinely internalized. New chaplains drown fastest when they're handed every edge case on day one instead of a single solid foundation.

***Days 31-60: Independent Practice With Close Feedback***

By day thirty, a new chaplain should be charting independently, but their notes should still be reviewed weekly, not just skimmed. This is the window where fixer language is easiest to catch and correct, before it calcifies into habit. Run the fifteen-minute audit from earlier in this chapter together, out loud, at least twice during this period. Ask the four self-assessment questions from Chapter Seven as a standing agenda item in supervision. This is also the right window to introduce IDG reporting expectations directly, coaching the new chaplain on translating their spiritual assessment into language the rest of the team can act on, the way Scenario H demonstrated.

### *Days 61-90: Consolidation and Peer Accountability*

By the end of the first ninety days, a new chaplain's documentation should be reviewed on the same rhythm as every other chaplain on your team, not singled out anymore as a new hire. This is the point to fold them into whatever peer accountability structure your team maintains, whether that's a monthly seminar, a chart-swap rhythm, or a formal verbatim group. If your team doesn't yet have that structure, a new chaplain's ninetieth day is as good a moment as any to build it, since onboarding naturally raises documentation to the front of everyone's mind anyway.

None of this requires much additional budget. It requires a leader who has decided documentation formation deserves the same seriousness as clinical competency in any other discipline, and who builds that seriousness into the calendar rather than hoping it happens organically. It rarely does, left to chance.

# Using This Book With a Team

If you're a hospice leader, a CPE supervisor, or a chaplaincy team lead reading this with an eye toward group formation, each chapter in this book ends with a short reflection section built for exactly that purpose. Work through one chapter per meeting with your team or cohort, using the reflection questions as discussion prompts rather than assigning the whole book at once. Documentation formation, like every other kind of pastoral formation, sticks best in small doses, discussed honestly in community, over time, not absorbed all at once and forgotten by the next hard week.

**FOR REFLECTION**

- *Where would this checklist live so you would actually see it before closing a note — your badge, your car dashboard, the inside cover of your work bag?*
- *Does your agency have a written chaplaincy documentation policy? If not, who is the right person for you to raise that conversation with this quarter?*

# Chapter 10
# A Closing Charge — Chart Like It Matters

I told you in the opening chapter that Jacob got his blessing and kept his limp, both at once, and I want to close this book by returning to that image, because it's the truest way I know to describe what I'm asking of you.

Charting well, over a long career, will not heal every wound this work leaves in you. You'll still carry some of the weight of the deaths you sat through, the families you couldn't fully comfort, the notes you wish you'd written differently on the hardest days. That weight isn't a sign you're doing this wrong. It's the cost of doing it at all, faithfully, as an actual human being rather than a detached technician. But good documentation, I've come to believe, is one of the quiet blessings available to us inside that cost. Not a cure for the limp. A way of making sure the walk wasn't wasted.

When you write a note that names what you saw, what was said, what you did, and what happened next, you aren't just completing a task. You're making sure the specific, unrepeatable soul you sat with doesn't disappear from the record the way so much of our own private grief disappears, unrecorded, into the years.

One thing to leave you with. Charting isn't the tax we pay for the privilege of doing real ministry at the bedside. It isn't administrative drudgery bolted onto the sacred work. It's the written form of sitting at the bedside. It is the only part of your presence that keeps sitting there, in the record, long after you've driven home for the evening.

When you write a note that names what you saw, what was said, what you did, and what happened next, you've extended your presence into every future hour that patient spends in this system, whether or not you're physically there to witness it. The nurse who reads your note inherits your presence. The social worker who reads it next week inherits your presence. The bereavement counselor who reads it after the funeral inherits your presence. That is one of the truest expressions of pastoral faithfulness available to us in this electronic age — the discipline of writing so well, so honestly, and so specifically that the patient's story survives us in the room, ready to be picked up by whoever comes next.

This book began with Jacob at the Jabbok, blessed and limping in the same sunrise, and every chapter since has tried to write from inside that same tension rather than resolve it prematurely for you. I'm not offering you a documentation system that will make hospice chaplaincy painless.

What I am offering is a way of carrying the weight of this work that doesn't lose the specific, unrepeatable people you've been entrusted with along the way. A way of walking with a limp that still, somehow, leaves a clear and faithful trail behind you for others to follow.

I think often about James, the surviving spouse from Scenario A and Scenario G, sitting in a too-quiet house three weeks after Helen's death, telling a chaplain on the phone that his prayers feel like talking to the ceiling. I made him up, in the sense that no specific James exists on any specific chart. But I've sat with a hundred variations of James, and I'll sit with a hundred more before I'm done with this work, and so will you. What James needed, in that moment, wasn't a chaplain with better theology than his grief could withstand. He needed a chaplain who'd been paying attention long enough, and writing carefully enough, to know exactly what had shifted in him since Helen died, and to say so plainly, without flinching from the fact that his faith currently felt like an empty room. That is what good documentation makes possible, across an entire length of stay and often for months into bereavement. Not a cure for the emptiness. A witness to it, faithful enough to notice when it starts, faithful enough to notice when something new begins to grow in its place.

Go back to your caseload this week and pick one thing from this book, just one, and try it on your very next note. Not all ten chapters. One. Then the next note, try another. That's how formation actually works, in documentation as in everything else. Not all at once, but faithfully, one note at a time, for as long as you're given to do this work.

Chart like it matters. Because it does.

**FOR REFLECTION**

- *What is the one thing from this book you will try on your very next chart note?*
- *Ten years from now, what do you want a chaplain who never met you to be able to learn about your ministry, purely from the record you left behind in the charts you wrote?*

# A Word to Hospice Leaders

If you lead a hospice organization, a spiritual care department, or a CPE program, a word directly to you before you hand this book to your chaplains, because what you do with it after that matters as much as anything written in the preceding ten chapters.

Documentation culture is a leadership issue, not merely an individual skill issue. I've consulted with agencies where a single excellent chaplain produced beautiful, clinically rich notes while three colleagues on the same team produced "Provided chaplaincy care" on a loop, and no one in leadership had ever named the gap, let alone addressed it. That gap isn't primarily a training failure. It's usually a leadership failure — an absence of a stated expectation, a documentation audit process, or a feedback loop that treats chaplaincy notes with the same seriousness leadership treats nursing or social work documentation. If you want the theology and the habits in this book to actually take root on your team, they need three things from you specifically: a chosen, consistent documentation model communicated clearly at orientation and reinforced afterward; a regular, low-stakes documentation review process (the fifteen-minute audit in Chapter Nine scales beautifully to a team setting) built into your existing supervision rhythm; and your own visible respect for the discipline, communicated not just in policy but in how you talk about spiritual care documentation in IDG, in team meetings, and in your own conversations with surveyors and auditors.

Protect time, too, for exactly the kind of peer accountability described in Chapter Seven. Chaplains, more than almost any other discipline on a hospice team, tend to work in relative isolation, one chaplain covering a wide territory with minimal direct oversight of their actual bedside or documentation practice. That isolation is structurally built into our field, and it's precisely the condition under which both excellent, quietly heroic ministry and slow, undetected burnout tend to happen without anyone else seeing either one clearly. A monthly seminar, a peer chart review, a documentation audit built into supervision — these aren't administrative luxuries. They are, in the language of Chapter One, systems of grace: structures that let good documentation, and good pastoral care, survive your chaplains' hardest weeks rather than depending entirely on their best ones.

Thank you for leading well enough to be reading a book like this one at all. That instinct, to invest in your chaplains' formation rather than simply assuming it will happen on its own, is itself a form of the hesed this whole book has been describing.

# About the Author

Dr. Bobby Bressman, D.Min., CGP, is a hospice chaplain, pastor, and author who serves as Regional Manager of Bereavement across a multi-state hospice organization, where he trains and supervises chaplains in clinical documentation, spiritual assessment, and bereavement care. He is the founder of GriefBites and the Grief2Growth Foundation, a ministry built at the intersection of faith and loss, offering Christ-centered resources to individuals in grief, pastors and churches, hospice organizations, and grieving leaders. He is currently completing CPEI training toward Board Certified Chaplain Educator and Supervisor credentialing.

Bobby's work is shaped by his own experience of deep personal loss, pastoral trauma; and burnout. That is the "limp" he leads from, and the conviction underneath every page of this book that our wounds, offered honestly, can become systems of grace for others. He and the GriefBites team build practical, theologically grounded tools for chaplains, churches, and hospice teams, including the RESTORE Pathway diagnostic suite, CE and CPEI training resources for chaplains, and B2B compliance and documentation resources for hospice organizations.

To learn more about GriefBites, access companion resources to this book, or invite Dr. Bressman to speak or train your team, visit GriefBites.org.

Companion resources referenced throughout this book — including a printable Charting Checklist, a Phrases That Help and Phrases That Hurt reference card, and a Sample Documentation Policy Template your agency can adapt — are available through GriefBites.org for individual chaplains, CPE cohorts, and hospice organizations.

www.ingramcontent.com/pod-product-compliance
Lightning Source LLC
LaVergne TN
LVHW060454061126
851857LV00016B/1827